T0300038

ROUTLEDGE LIBRARY EDITIONS:
THE ADOLESCENT

Volume 13

AIDS AND ADOLESCENTS

AIDS AND ADOLESCENTS

Edited by
LORRAINE SHERR

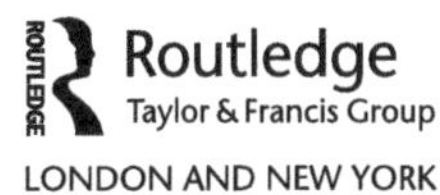

LONDON AND NEW YORK

First published in 1997 by Harwood Academic Publishers

This edition first published in 2023
by Routledge
4 Park Square, Milton Park, Abingdon, Oxon OX14 4RN

and by Routledge
605 Third Avenue, New York, NY 10158

Routledge is an imprint of the Taylor & Francis Group, an informa business

ISBN: 978-1-032-37655-4 (Set)
ISBN: 978-1-032-39831-0 (Volume 13) (hbk)
ISBN: 978-1-032-39873-0 (Volume 13) (pbk)
ISBN: 978-1-003-35178-8 (Volume 13) (ebk)

DOI: 10.4324/9781003351788

Publisher's Note
The publisher has gone to great lengths to ensure the quality of this reprint but points out that some imperfections in the original copies may be apparent.

Disclaimer
The publisher has made every effort to trace copyright holders and would welcome correspondence from those they have been unable to trace.

AIDS and Adolescents

Edited by
Lorraine Sherr
University of London, UK

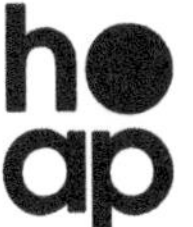

harwood academic publishers
Australia • Canada • China • France • Germany • India
Japan • Luxembourg • Malaysia • The Netherlands • Russia
Singapore • Switzerland • Thailand • United Kingdom

Published in The Netherlands by Harwood Academic Publishers.

Printed in India.

Amsteldijk 166
1st Floor
1079 LH Amsterdam
The Netherlands

British Library Cataloguing in Publication Data

Aids and adolescents
1. Aids (Disease) in adolescence 2. Teenagers – Sexual behaviour 3. Aids (Disease) in adolescence – Social aspects
I. Sherr, Lorraine
362.1'9'69792'00835

ISBN 90-5702-039-4

To my mother
Billy (Lilian) Isaacs,
Aunty Joy, Aunty Fanyse
and
Carmel College

Contents

Acknowledgements

Any compilation of work represents input and help from a wide range of people. Many of the issues came to fruition in the course of a number of studies, which I would like to note particularly. These are the EC funded studies on Ante-natal Testing in HIV Infection, the multinational Scenario Analysis and the AIDS, Discrimination and Legal Services study. I would like to acknowledge the help of Elaine Harris who worked tirelessly, and Janis Hodges and Anna Bergenstrom who facilitated the work. My own adolescents put some of the thinking straight by their knowing comments – thanks to Ari, Ilan, Yoni and Liora.

Gail Goldburg spent much time on the proofs and index. Her wonderful support is gratefully acknowledged. Adele and Trevot kept us distracted and Benjamin Whine took on all catering.

Contributors

PETER AGGLETON
Director
Thomas Coram Research Unit, Institute of Education, University of London, London, UK

STEPHANE BLANCHE
Professeur de Universities Practicien, Hospitalier
Department de Pediatrie, Hospital Necker-Enfants Malades, Paris, France

GLYNIS M. BREAKWELL
Pro Vice Chancellor (of University)
Social Psychology European, Research Institute, University of Surrey, Guildford, UK

JUNE CRAWFORD
Research Consultant
National Centre for HIV Social, Research, Macquarie University, Australia

RICHARD CURTIS
Research Consultant
John Jay College, New York City, USA

MARIANNE DEBRE
Medecin des Hospitaux
Hospital Necker-Enfants Malades, Paris, France

RALPH J. DICLEMENTE
Professor Dept. of Health Behaviour, Dept. of Paediatrics, Dept. of Medicine, Associate Dir. Centre for AIDS Research
University of Alabama, Birmingham, Alabama, USA

HAFTAN M. ECKHOLDT
Assistant Professor
Dept of Psychiatry, Dept of Preventive Medicine & Community Health, New Jersey Medical School, New Jersey, USA

JONATHAN ELFORD
Senior Lecturer in Epidemiology
Dept of Primary Care & Population, Sciences, Royal Free Hospital, London, UK

SAMUEL R. FRIEDMAN
Doctor
Narcotic and Drug Research, National Development & Institute Inc, New York, USA

ISABELLE FUNCK-BRENTANO
Clinical Psychologist
Department de Pediatrie, Hospital Necker-Enfants Malades, Paris, France

STEPHEN R. HOOPER
Associate Professor in Psychiatry
Clinical Centre for the Study of Development and Learning University of North Carolina School of Medicine, USA

DON C. DES JARLAIS
Professor Research Consultant
Beth Israel Medical Centre, New York, USA

VALERIE JOHNSON
Research Consultant
Rutgers University, New Brunswick, New Jersey, USA

BENNY JOSE
Research Consultant
National Development & Research Institute, New York, New Jersey, USA

CHERYL ANN KENNEDY
Assistant Professor
Dept of Psychiatry, Dept of Preventive Medicine & Community Health, New Jersey Medical School, Newark, USA

SUSAN KIPPAX
Director
National Centre in HIV Social Research, Macquarie University, New South Wales, Australia

RICHARD LOVELY
Research Consultant
Battelle Seattle Research Centre, Seattle, USA

GENE A. MCGRADY
Research Consultant
Morehouse School of Medicine, Atlanta, GA USA

LORRAINE SHERR
Senior Lecturer Health Psychology
Dept of Primary Care & Population Sciences, Royal Free Hospital London, UK

FLORENCE VEBER
Medecin des Hopitaux
Department de Pediatrie, Hospital Necker-Enfants Malades, Paris, France

MILDRED VERA
Research Consultant
University of Puerto Rico, Medical Sciences Campus, San Juan, Puerto Rico, USA

IAN WARWICK
Assistant Director Health & Education Research Unit
Institute of Education University of London, London, UK

HELENE R. WHITE
Research Consultant
Rutgers University, New Brunswick, New Jersey, USA

ALAN NEAIGUS
Research Consultant
Narcotic & Drug Research, National Development & Research Institutes Inc. New York, USA

DENISE PAONE
Research Consultant
Beth Israel Medical Centre, New York, USA

BARRY S. PETERS
Senior Lecturer & Head of Academic Dept
Genitourinary Medicine & HIV, United Medical Schools of Guy's & St. Thomas' Hospital, London, UK

ANN REID
Research Registrar in GU, Medicine & Medical Education
United Medical Schools of Guy's & St. Thomas' Hospital, London UK

DOREEN ROSENTHAL
Director
Centre for the Study of Transmissible Diseases, La Trobe University, Melbourne, Australia

J. KENNETH WHITT
Associate Professor Dept Psychiatry
Department of Psychiatry & Pediatrics, University of North Carolina, School of Medicine, USA

JONATHAN ZENILMAN
Research Consultant
Johns Hopkins University, New Brunswick, New Jersey, USA

1

Introduction

LORRAINE SHERR

There is something exhilarating about the hope and challenge that the young add to any debate. It is timely that a long hard look at adolescents in the arena of HIV and AIDS feeds the dialogue. This text on adolescents provides an insight into a wide range of adolescent issues which are rarely compiled in the literature, let alone pursued. Much of the HIV epidemic response has been at the individual level in the hope that this narrow focus will provide the key to containment and resolution of spread. However, over ten years after the epidemic has taken hold, it is clear that paradigms are limited, input is uncritical and large cohorts are overlooked. In this text a series of contributions have been compiled to explore adolescent issues ranging from sexual behaviour, health education campaigns, HIV prevention and HIV/AIDS care.

In the first chapter, I provide an overview of adolescent problems and why they are so often overlooked or submerged. A clear understanding of whether they do indeed differ, and if so in what ways is urgently needed. The chapter goes on to explore the countless studies on students and their utility, issues such as adolescent sexual behaviour and condom use and moves on to key challenges around HIV testing and adolescents. Sexual abuse is a common phenomenon and new infection in the young may mark tomorrow's epidemic. The chapter explores a wide range of issues such as gay and bisexual youth, youth with haemophilia, pregnancy, homeless and runaway teenagers, and gender, and culminates in a section examining the psychological factors associated with HIV positive youth and those with AIDS. This covers mental health reactions, care, orphans, bereavement, ethics and rights and family issues. This chapter is followed by a comprehensive epidemiological analysis by Elford who provides up to date HIV and AIDS surveillance with particular focus on Europe generally and the UK specifically to point out the nuances of seroprevalence and incidence surveys and the implications these may have for future action and data gathering. This chapter is followed by a chapter on AIDS diagnosis in US adolescents by Kennedy and Eckholdt who then provide an insight into where they see the future. They provide epidemiology with insights into age, race, racial distribution, gender ratio, transmission group and social backdrop in order to explore policy implications.

Kippax and Crawford provide a fascinating challenge about the facts and fictions associated with adolescent risk. They explore incidence and prevalence and predictors of seroconversion with an insight into behaviour of homosexually active men and heterosexual students. They critically examine risk among the young, correlates of such risk and proceed to comment on ethnicity, homelessness, interpersonal skills and gender/sexual identity issues. This chapter may challenge some of the basic notions underpinning many approaches and may help workers reformulate and refocus some of their efforts. The following chapter by Aggleton and Warwick provides insightful example of some of the issues raised by Kippax and Crawford as they explore young people, sexuality and HIV/AIDS education. They challenge some of the meaningful versus rhetorical health promotion efforts and provide an overview of approaches from school based to out of school approaches as well as focused insights. Rosenthal's chapter then proceeds to provide insight on expanding this context. This study of Australian adolescents' behaviours and beliefs about HIV/AIDS and other STDs may well provide a model for many explorations across the world. She examines sexual practices, knowledge and places HIV in the context of STD's generally. She provides insight into sources of information such as parents, peers and others and looks at attitudes to AIDS prevention strategies, perceptions of risk and attempts to construct sexuality beliefs and competencies. The chapter goes on to explore some sexual myths, masculinity and femininity issues and confidence and communication. All these are relevant to the way in which adolescents construct a sexual identity and are discussed in the light of the HIV epidemic.

Drug injection is a particular issue for adolescents and Friedman *et al.* (chapter 7) provide a comprehensive overview of this issue from an American perspective. The study explores the rates of infection with HIV and other agents which can be transmitted via drug injection and sex. They examine how heterosexual youth come to be at risk for HIV via their drug or sexual networks and then go on to explore predictors of problem substance use and problem behaviour. This chapter then proceeds to examine personal characteristics, interpersonal factors and wider sociodemographic factors in substance use. Finally they put forward some of the recent findings on the sexual networks of adolescence. Breakwell provides a chapter exploring adolescents and emerging sexuality. She challenges whether this is truly emerging or rather continuing and explores the lexicon of sexuality, sexual identities, preoccupations and self efficacy. This gives rise to comment on risk taking and vulnerability.

The chapters then provide a more focused view on those with HIV infection. Hooper and Whitt provide an overview of adolescents facing AIDS and haemophilia with a review of current findings, neuropsychological factors and psychosocial issues. This overview provides some comment on emerging issues and future directions. Funk Brentano et al provide an insightful look at adaptation and coping of HIV infected adolescents living in France. They pay particular attention to cognitive development, school achievement and psychological adjustment. They explore in depth the emotional needs of such adolescents with an examination of issues of disclosure and adolescent's perceptions of the disease. This is supplemented by a chapter from Peters examining the medical management of AIDS in adolescents with a useful overview of issues, current approaches and problems due to the paucity of adolescent data. Finally the text ends with a chapter from DiClemente examining future directions for prevention of HIV among adolescents.

This compilation of chapters is aimed at providing an overview of the many facets of adolescence and HIV issues. It is an attempt to encompass a variety of perspectives, approaches, points of view and, at times, disparate areas. Some workers approach contentious issues, such as health education, from critical perspectives. The way forward must be to gain an overview of the vast range of current thinking and utilise this in efforts to formulate future pathways. As the role of adolescence in the future of the HIV epidemic grows in focus the data base will widen and more comprehensive issues will emerge.

2

Adolescents and HIV in our Midst

LORRAINE SHERR

"SOCIETY HAS THE TEENAGERS IT DESERVES" (J.B. PRIESTLY) BUT DO TEENAGERS HAVE THE SOCIETY THEY DESERVE?

Caught in the cleft between paediatrics and adults, adolescents are often overlooked, underestimated, or ignored. They are too old to be children and too young to be adults and they are simply neglected in much of the literature. Traditionally adolescence is seen as a time of development deserving special attention. Although there is a controversy as to whether adolescence truly represents a time of storm and stress, it is certainly a time with different issues, challenges and dilemmas in the HIV field. There is a growing acknowledgement that the natural history of HIV may differ in various groups and this is worthy of individual study. Such knowledge may also help evaluation interventions as well as coping resources. For example Rosenberg *et al.*, (1994) have noted an age specific relative risk of progression from HIV seroconversion to AIDS onset. The disregard of adolescents is stark in the literature. There are countless studies which question people on the intricacies of their sexual behaviour, the exact point at which condoms are used, yet never bother to ask their ages. Often sex worker studies fail to elaborate if there are adolescents in their cohorts. Military recruits may well be in their teens, but again studies rarely differentiate between the 17 year olds and the adults. The same is true of countless drug user studies and gay men cohorts.

This chapter will initially explore the challenge of adolescents, how they are identified, the psychosocial studies that have been carried out and the understanding that exists of their particular role and problem. The next major theme to be tackled in this chapter is the psychological needs and responses to adolescents infected or affected directly by HIV. This will necessitate an overview of lessons learned about adolescents or pointers from other areas which may be of use to adolescents. It will also explore some of the notions associated with Adolescents and HIV such as care issues, bereavement and loss, orphan issues and the emerging focus groups which may need particular attention and monitoring. Finally some evaluation of ethics and rights will be explored as they affect the mental health needs of adolescents with HIV issues in their life.

NATURE OF ADOLESCENCE AND ADOLESCENT SEXUALITY

The recognition and description of adolescence as a distinct phase is a relatively recent phenomenon (Shaffer 1995) and many of the concepts do not have the same meaning in different cultural contexts. Adolescence is usually heralded by physical changes and sexual maturity as well as a variety of emotional and developmental challenges. Some define adolescents by those in the teenage years, others define it by a stage of development of maturity. In general there is no clear definition of adolescents and the term is often used interchangeably with youth. For the purpose of this text the interim phase between childhood and adulthood will be concentrating on the teenage years with an acknowledgement that younger teenagers may differ significantly with older teenagers, and that in some cultures age related roles and expectations differ dramatically.

Adolescent sexuality is an important factor in any study of HIV and these issues are discussed at length in the chapter by Breakwell (chapter 8). Studies of teenage sexuality have noted a variety of changes over time with earlier menarche, the infiltration and change to global media and insight into different cultures, there is an increased urbanisation which can account for change as can increases in poverty, social constraints are easing and more girls in the world are attending school. Age at first sex varies in studies across the world (Botswana 17.3 years, Cameroon 16.1 years, Indonesia 19.8 years, Mexico 19.8 years, Paraguey 18.9 years, USA 16.1 years). Similarly studies which explore childbirth by the age of 20 can reveal trends of adolescent sexual behaviour ranging from 75% in Nigeria to 30% in the USA. Sexual violence also seems to be a reality documented in teenage sexual development.

ADOLESCENTS – ARE THEY THERE?

The silence of data on HIV positive adolescents may indeed make people overlook their existence. There are a number of reasons why their profile may be low. If they are contained within other subgroups they are simply subsumed with scant recognition of the fact that a young gay positive adolescent may have dramatically different needs to an adult. Similarly a young drug user may be blurred among the cohort.

The group of children acquiring HIV through vertical transmission are young because of the relative newness of the epidemic rather than that they do not or will not emerge as adolescents. There are clear indications from the studies that survival into adolescents is possible, probable and potential. For example van den Berg *et al.*, (1994) followed up a small cohort of 11 children ten years after HIV infection from plasma donation. Three of the children died within the first two and a half years of life, five others died between 6.2 and 11 years after infection and three survived. The data explored in detail their immunoglobulin levels, disease severity, volume of transfused plasma and age at transfusion. However, little data was gathered on the emotional traumas on these young children and how they adapted and coped with HIV disease. It is clear if workers do not track the psychosocial aspects of HIV in this emerging population any attempts to intervene, ameliorate suffering or aide coping will be delayed by the lack of insight and systematic evaluation.

Few national studies are carried out. Kaplan & Schonberg (1994) pointed to adolescent overviews in the USA and noted that they comprised only 1% of the total number of individuals reported with AIDS. However, a sensitive examination of the time trends in this group reveals a rapid increase in cases which may merit particular attention.

Another way to hide adolescents is simply to make them grow up. For example in many African population studies it is hard to find if any adolescents are included. This is clarified by some studies which rob adolescents of their rights. Mulder *et al.*, (1994) carried out a study of mortality in 15 villages in Uganda over a 2 year period. HIV data was available for 9389 individuals and prevalence of HIV was found at 4.8% for all ages and 8.2% for adults. They classify adults as those aged 13 or more.

Adolescents are also veiled by the failure to explore the implications of the very figures in front of everyone's eyes. It is known that a high proportion of people with AIDS are diagnosed in their twenties. It is also known that the incubation period of HIV can be many years. If these two figures are conflated then it seems reasonable to assume that a great many people diagnosed with disease in their twenties probably became HIV positive as adolescents. HIV incidence figures usually reflects testing policy rather than true prevalence. AIDS figures are much more reliable and should be used for a retrospective look at the position of adolescents in the infection rates.

Yet another to conceal adolescents is simply to ignore them in poor countries. For example D' Angelo (1994) reporting on the "epidemiology of AIDS in adolescents" reports USA figures only in such a way as to overlook the rest of the world, such as "as of June 30, 1993, 913 cases of AIDS among adolescents 13-19 years old had been reported to the CDC". Thus international texts on paediatric HIV overlook adolescents in the remainder of the world and the fact that it is a relatively small problem in the richer centres does not mean it is globally unproblematic.

Finally of 220 studies identified via a Medline computer search on AIDS and adolescents over 1994-1995, only five of them examined adolescents with HIV infection or living in a home with others (siblings or parents) who were HIV positive or who had died from an AIDS related illness. The remainder of the studies explored attitudes, behaviour, thoughts, feelings, opinions, judgements, views, comments and confessions of teenagers across the globe. Their repetitiveness and lack of progression were distressing.

ADOLESCENTS – DO THEY DIFFER?

There is evidence that survival times and types of disease differ between adults and children (Turner *et al.*, 1995). Median survival times after AIDS diagnosis, for example in the above study was 62 months for all children compared with 11 months for adults. Many of the studies on adolescents are concentrated among groups who also have haemophilia. This is problematic in terms of generalisation of findings. For a start if infection can be dated to a specific blood transfusion these cohorts may well differ from those infected vertically given that their early development was not in the presence of HIV. Ramafedi and Lauer (1995) examined survival trends in HIV positive adolescents who were not haemophiliacs (n=117) and found that 14% died of AIDS related conditions. The survival time for this group from diagnosis of HIV was 3 years. Cumulative survival for the cohort at 8 years after diagnosis was 52% with a median observation time range of 4 years, irrespective of gender, race and mode of transmission factors.

HIV and AIDS may not be the foremost concern for sexually active adolescents. Klussman *et al.* (1993) found in a survey of behaviour attitudes and AIDS concerns in 687 adolescents in Germany that pregnancy was a greater worry than AIDS for most young people. Risk and its perception is discussed in detail in chapters 4, 5 and 6. Studies have shown that adolescents knowledge about HIV is only weakly related to behaviour (Brown *et al.*, 1991, Pontal *et al.*, 1991) with a wide range of issues affecting views on safe behaviour such as condom use (Brown *et al.*, 1992).

Some adolescents differ on the very axes which are used to explore HIV, its prevention and its transmission. For example it is well documented that adolescent drug users are less likely to be present in treatment centres and thus less likely to be monitored in studies or to be the recipients of interventions based on harm reduction in drug use. This despite the fact that there is good evidence that much drug and alcohol use commences in adolescent years.

GENDER ISSUES AND ADOLESCENTS

Although gender has been seen as a vital issue in understanding adult HIV infection, it is invariably simply overlooked in children and adolescents. This is odd, given that gender does not simply become an issue as one enters adulthood, but plays an important part in the development of the child and emerging adolescent. Few studies that explore adolescent issues in AIDS also hold the problems of gender in the balance. Indeed Forsyth (1995) reports that in the USA some population groups report higher infection rates among females than males. Behaviour and behaviour change may also be gender related. Traditional care roles may disproportionately revert to female children and gender issues in emerging sexuality may be of particular importance. Some studies (Chen *et al.*, 1991, Squire 1993) have explored the tendency of older men to take younger women as sexual partners as an HIV avoidance strategy. Clearly such behaviour has implications for adolescent women which need exploring.

STUDENTS – TOO MUCH STUDY AND TOO LITTLE APPLICATION

It is sad to note that much of the literature on adolescents reported in the academic journals is a random gathering of pen and paper studies exploring in depth university and high school student's views. Although this may have been helpful, even vital, in the early days of the epidemic – the utility of such studies is now questionable given that the international community rarely used these studies as the basis of sound programmes. The course of HIV spread is also often tracked in communities who are rarely studied in terms of their behaviour and attitudes. The disproportionate numbers of reported studies on attitudes and sexual behaviour in university students compared to the natural history and tracking of HIV in positive adolescents is distressing.

The studies are often similar. They rarely use sound methodology. Indeed in a recent review (Oakley, 1995) out of many studies few identified met the methodological criteria for evaluation. Attitude studies are rarely linked to HIV status. The few studies which do this reveal some interesting findings. For example, Raab *et al.*, studied 4,665 students who were tested for HIV. Five tested positive, all from the highest risk group (1.2 per 10,000 for all respondents). Factors associated with positivity were residence in Africa, IDU and homosexuality.

ADOLESCENT SEXUAL BEHAVIOUR AND CONDOM USE

Sexually transmitted diseases have long been a problem for adolescents. Indeed Forsyth (1995) reports that "every year, one of every eight sexually active adolescents in infected with a sexually transmitted disease". The area of attitudes and behaviour around sexual behaviour is probably the most studied area in relation to HIV and adolescents, despite backlash from those who fear that condom promotion would initiate first sex or sexual behaviour which fears are essentially unfounded (Sellers *et al.*, 1994).

Magura *et al.*, (1994) studied condom use in 421 sexually active minority male adolescents serving in jail within New York City. Prior to arrest multiple sexual partners were commonly reported as was anal intercourse (33% of the sample). Regular condom use was rare, with inconsistency normative. 17% never used condoms. AIDS education in jail could be an interesting innovation.

Patterns of sexual behaviour have been studied in a number of centres, where youth have been included. For example Konings *et al.*, examined a sample in Tanzania and found that age of first intercourse was 15 years or younger and concluded that more recent birth cohorts have behaviour patterns that increase the risk of sexually transmitted infectious agents as behaviour patterns change over time. Maxwell *et al.*, (1995) reported some interesting findings in decision making in a cohort of adolescent STD attenders in California. Essentially, condom use with regular partners was low (3.8%) and inconsistent with casual partners (36%). They found that decision making for using condoms reflected different pathways than decisions not to use. Not to use condoms was often a joint decision, whereas utilisation was seen as an individual decision in this study.

McCabe reported on a relationship between syphilis seropositivity and HIV infection in a sample of 59 adolescents (McCabe *et al.*, 1993). A number of studies have explored risk behaviour among adolescent groups (Moscicki *et al.*, 1993; Orr & Langefeld, 1993). Keller (1993) attempted to advance an understanding of the risk taking in young adults by exploring the mental schema they constructed around HIV infection and linking this to problems they may have in using and initiating condoms. This study showed that schema need to be complete if condoms are to be used successfully. This was not found and gaps in schematic knowledge were supplemented by problems with condom use resulting in a low uptake of systematic condom use.

Many studies focus simply on condom use despite the need to explore issues beyond condoms in terms of HIV prevention. Levy *et al.*, (1993) showed that adolescents responded differently to safe sex issues compared to drug issues in their appraisal of willingness to discuss the topic, to divulge their behaviour to their parents or their ability to refuse drugs.

One of the problems with HIV and adolescents has been this condom narrowness. Theoretical and analytical models that extend beyond the hard sell of condoms to the young are few and far between. In years to come workers may question the wisdom and utility of this narrow approach (Reid, 1995).

HIV TESTING AND ADOLESCENTS

Do adolescents differ from adults? What does differ is the fact that their opinions are rarely sought. Rawitscher *et al.* (1995) explored preferences regarding HIV testing expounded by adolescents and found that they preferred to be tested by someone who did not know them and they also preferred doctors to initiate the discussions about HIV related risk behaviours.

There is often a push to test those who have limited abilities to consent fully. Such examples are pregnant women, prisoners etc. It will be worrying if this trend extends to adolescents.

Goodman *et al.* (1994) note "perseverance pays off". In a study of high risk adolescent girls set up to explore use of confidential HIV testing services they noted that a significant proportion of high risk adolescent girls were willing to utilise services.

A cohort of 2,548 adolescents in the USA were examined comparing the 11.5%

who had undergone HIV antibody testing with those 88.5% who had not. Those reporting HIV testing were more often male, black, urban dwellers, injection drug users and more sexually active - commencing at an earlier age and reporting more partners. Despite these global differences, in depth analyses revealed that over half of the tested group reported no HIV risks whilst a quarter of adolescents not tested had at least one identifiable risk factor.

Can adolescents give informed consent and what are the pre and post test counselling restrictions which should emanate the Futterman and Hein (1994) report on five key principles for adolescent HIV counselling which include:

i. Developmentally and culturally appropriate pre and post test HIV counselling.

ii. Those capable of consent should be allowed to give it

iii. Testing should be voluntary

iv. Confidentiality is important

v. Access to treatment (and research) should be available.

Although these notions are lofty, their practicality and the extent to which they are applied can be questioned. It may be difficult to derive clear guidance on how one would measure whether an adolescent is capable of consent and what elements constitute a lack of such capability. Confidentiality cannot be guaranteed if informed consent is not met. The situation is further compounded when adolescents are seen in a family clinic and their needs may be subsumed within the family need or the preexisting relationship the family has with the care setting.

The current emphasis on HIV testing in ante-natal clinics must also take adolescents into account. Given the high rate of adolescent pregnancy and the particularly difficult issues associated with ante-natal HIV diagnosis, such testing should never be routine and should always include an informed dialogue with the adolescents themselves.

SEXUAL ABUSE AND ADOLESCENT HIV

Sexual abuse has always been a potential contributor to HIV transmission and there have been cases where abuse has been recorded as the most likely source of infection (Sherr *et al.*, 1993; Murphy *et al.*, 1989; Claydon *et al.*, 1991). Abuse is often, though not always, directed at the young. Indeed there are oft noted cycles of behaviour which emanate in or result from abuse, which enhance the possibility of risk exposure. For example abuse may lead to drug use or vice versa.

HIV testing protocols are needed to inform practice when dealing with young people who have been sexually abused (Sherr, 1995). In a study of 28 children Durfee (1995) explored the needs of such children. Gellert *et al.*, (1993) noted that 4.1% of a clinic population had become infected through sexual abuse. Gutman (1994) notes that the true number of children infected via sexual abuse is unknown, and the numbers which do exist are probably underestimations given the barriers to reporting and the difficulties in diagnosis. Garcia (1995) noted that 1.7% of paediatric HIV cases seen in Mexico had associated abuse documented. Lindegren (1995) reported on a nationwide study in the USA where 6 cases of sexual abuse were noted as the means of HIV transmission in young people from a sample set of 4,903. This generates a 0.2% rate – lower than the Mexican study. All the perpetrators of abuse in this study were male. Very few studies exist documenting this potentially enormous problem. However, Stevens (1995) noted a high rate of HIV and STDs in children evacuated from war zones in Sierra Leone. Di John (1990) recorded two case histories where sexual abuse was probably implicated in transmission, and Caselli (1989) reports adolescent abuse as a route of infection.

NEW INFECTION IN THE YOUNG – TOMORROW'S EPIDEMIC?

Young gay men in San Francisco were becoming infected at a rate of 2.6% per year (Osmond *et al.*, 1994) despite the fact that they became sexually active after awareness of AIDS was widespread. Maxwell *et al.* (1995) explored the prevalence of high risk behaviours in teenagers attending STD clinics in the USA. Males reported earlier commencement of sexual activity than females (14 years vs 14.9 years in this study). Consistent condom use was rare with steady partners, and incomplete with casual partners.

Some behaviour changes that are noted among older men is a tendency to seek out younger (and thus HIV free) female sexual partners. However, for those younger women, invariably adolescents, this brings with it a risk of infection.

Behaviour change is not simply a matter of health advertising. After a decade of the epidemic, one encounters a safe sex weary public and there is little new in the messages. Most adolescents of today have never known a world without HIV or AIDS.

GAY AND BISEXUAL YOUTH

There is a growing literature on a variety of aspects of sexuality, risk and adaptation in gay and bisexual men, but few explore age factors or focus specifically on youth. Bochow *et al* (1994) reported on an exhaustive study in 9 European centres of gay and bisexual men. They found that sexuality patterns were strikingly similar, but strategies of risk management varied considerably, irrespective of rates of reported HIV in the various communities (ranging from 7% to 17%). These authors note the importance of including gay and bisexual men in prevention campaigns. This may well apply all the more so for youth.

The few studies of young gay and bisexual men show worrying trends. In California a 425 subject study (Lemp *et al.*, 1994) revealed a seroprevalence of 9.4% nearly three quarters of whom did not know of thier own HIV status despite a wide range of risk behaviours catalogued. The new generational needs are posed as a challenge. A study of gay youth was conducted by Rotheram Borus *et al* (1994) in

New York. Intervention and one year follow up revealed reductions in unprotected same sex and oral acts. Partner number was reduced after intervention.

YOUTH WITH HAEMOPHILIA

Much of the understanding of HIV in adolescents comes from the group of teenagers with Haemophilia (Bor *et al.*, 1992), Goldsmith (1994). However, it is difficult to generalise from this cohort given the specific implications of a double disease and the preexisting care and management protocols which were set up around haemophilia services.

Hooper *et al.* (1993) found no evidence of behavioural problems in asymptomatic HIV seropositive adolescents with haemophilia when compared with HIV seronegative controls. Gertner et al. (1994) reported on an ongoing study of 300 boys with haemophilia of whom 62% were also HIV positive . HIV infection seemed to contribute to lowered weight, height and triceps skin fold thickness in this group.

Miller (1995) describes how HIV interrupts the adolescent's normal life stage and expectations. Relationships are often made difficult because of dual loyalties to the adolescent and to the parent. Issues that emerge in this account focus on the process of informing the adolescent about both HIV and haemophilia and how to hold the best interest of the child as paramount while balancing transmission and emotional risks.

HOMELESS AND RUNAWAY YOUTH

There is a growing body of literature documenting HIV prevalence or more noticeably risk behaviours in cohorts of homeless, runaway or street youth (see Lhuede & Moore; 1994, Turtle, 1994). These studies show a high level of risk yet it is always unclear whether the risk is a result of the social conditions or vice versa.

PREGNANT YOUTH

The single minded researchers subdivide this epidemic into compartments which aide and assist research, service delivery and understanding. Reality, however, is rarely neat and tidy. Teenage pregnancy is a fact and there is no reason to believe that HIV positive teenagers should differ in their pregnancy rates. Indeed there is every pointer that given the sexually transmitted nature of HIV, those more likely to become infected through exposure to risk may be more likely to conceive as well. Indeed, Levine (1995) points out that in the ACTG 076 trial of zidovudine in pregnancy, pregnant women participated in the study with an age range commencing at 15.

It is in this arena that many issues comes to the fore. The whole notion of HIV testing a pregnant teenager challenges the notions of informed consent, confidentiality and emotional support. The pregnant teenager, herself in need, must also take on the responsibility of the potentially HIV positive child. Adult studies rarely involve partners, yet for teenagers as well as adults this may be a shortcoming. If the pregnancy is allied to poverty, drug use, poor housing on unemployment, non-judgemental services need to be brought in.

HIV POSITIVE YOUTH

The passage of time will inevitably reveal growing numbers of adolescents living with HIV reflecting current and past vertical transmission. Grubman *et al.* (1995) described a cohort of children living with HIV beyond the age of 9 years. They found one quarter of the sample at this age to be asymptomatic, while the remainder had many symptoms which were chronic and impeded daily living. In a study of young women in Rwanda Bulterys *et al.* (1994) reported that teenage women were at the highest risk of HIV infection over a two year study period with infection rates highest among the poorer women. Sexual behaviour patterns were explored and the authors recommend intervention programmes for young teenagers prior to onset of sexual activity.

Forsyth (1995) reports that 0.2% of American college students were HIV positive and 1 in every 278 job corps applicants were HIV positive. These rates were higher in urban settings. Change over time also shows an alarming increase with 1 out of every 244 adolescent health clinic attenders testing HIV positive in a Washington study in 1987 and a five fold increase documented by 1992 to 1 in 52 (D' Angelo, 1992).

Hein *et al.* (1995) explored sexual and drug use as well as psychosocial issues with HIV positive adolescents and compared this cohort to a group of HIV negative adolescents. 72 HIV positive adolescents (age 13-21 years) were compared with 1142 negative. 11% more positive adolescents were identified in the cohort through blinded seroprevalence screening of the negative cohort. Sexual abuse rates were high for the cohort, but significantly raised in the HIV positive group (33 vs 21%). The ongoing risk behaviour of these HIV positive adolescents was notable. Both anal and survival sex were more common in the positives and this behaviour appeared to be current (32% vs 4%), unprotected sex was reported in 42% with casual partners, and sex was often in the presence of drugs (52%). All these behaviours were significantly more prevalent in the HIV positive group than the HIV negative group. Not surprisingly sexually transmitted diseases were common (59%) and multiple drug use was also reported by just under half the group.

Within the group the HIV positive females reported consistent different behaviour patterns compared to the HIV negative females with more oral and anal intercourse. Few theoretical models helped in predicting these behaviours, although themes of abuse history and homelessness were elaborated.

MENTAL HEALTH NEEDS OF HIV POSITIVE ADOLESCENTS.

Although there has been some advances in understanding medical care and management in paediatrics generally, and adolescents to some extent (Pizzo & Wilfert, 1994) the area of psychological effects is sorely neglected. Laryea and Gien (1993) point to loneliness, coping challenges, stigmatisation and disruptions in both family and peer relationships. They noted that their sample reported prolonged uncertainty and this generated intense and constant fear of their illness, of disclosure and of societal rejection. Such anxieties were often not aired.

It is unclear where understanding should commence. Studies from the adult literature point to a range of negative emotions such as anxiety, depression, suicide and panic attacks. There is a general acceptance that the issues for younger clients are not necessarily the same. Furthermore the paucity of studies makes generalisations and comprehensive understanding difficult if not impossible.

★ Extreme emotional reactions – Very few studies have documented the range of reactions. Futterman and Hein (1994) note that suicidal attempts did not increase after HIV positivity but suicidal ideation showed a minimal increase. This cross sectional study may be interesting to review over time. Anxiety and depression ought to be anticipated, but ways of expression and coping strategies may differ from both adult and younger child cohorts. Draimen *et al.* (1992) found no evidence of extreme anxiety in standardised measures on a group of adolescents but did note that youth commonly checked items of externalising symptoms. One must bear in mind that some of these paper and pen inventories may not be particularly sensitive to adolescent mood swings and this same study noted that over half of the adolescents were judged as clinically depressed.

★ Confidentiality – Adolescents may have particular problems with confidentiality and exerting control on who their status is divulged to. This is particularly true for those who were infected as young children. By the time they reach adolescents they cannot undo who has been told, even if they would not agree with it. Thus adolescents may be in a different position to adults and the same rules and constraints may not be relevant. Clearly for newly diagnosed adolescents confidentiality can be should be respected.

★ Curiosity – Adolescents may have many questions which become more sophisticated and intense with understanding. If an adolescent has been infected for a long period of time, workers may overlook their constant need for explanations, information and dialogue. Questioning, when paced, allows children to gather in information to meet their comprehension. It is important that when such children reach adolescence their curiosity is still encouraged and avenues for questions and answers are maintained.

★ Emerging sexuality – Emerging sexuality creates many burdens for the HIV positive youth with very few studies on their reactions, needs and behaviour. For many adolescents sexual exploration and relationship formation are intricately linked. HIV infection impedes both sexual development and may affect relationship plans and realities.

- Relationships – HIV may place a strain on youth in forming meaningful relationships. The barriers may be real or artificial and those who do have good peer relationships benefit from these.
- Self esteem – A sense of self and self esteem issues may well be critically questioned for adolescents with HIV infection (Borden, 1989).
- Behavioural problems – At times of stress or trauma, behavioural challenges may be a common pathway for the adolescent - with different forms emerging depending on age, social circumstance and environment. Draiman *et al.*, (1992) noted in a sample of 58 adolescents with HIV from 40 families that 34% were "acting out", 58% had shown a decline in school achievement linked to parental illness and a quarter of the boys in the study had problems with the law.
- Loss – Adolescents with AIDS or HIV infection are highly likely to have experienced loss. Draiman *et al.*, (1992) noted that on average the adolescents in their sample had experienced four major losses in the past two years and over 80% recorded at least one loss.
- End of Life issues – For adolescents the range of end of life issues are similar to adults. They too may experience suicidal ideation thoughts and acts. Suicide in general is increasing within adolescent groups across the world, and HIV should not be ignored as a potential trigger. Choice of means and place of death is often provided to adults and children's wishes should also be respected. Fears and thoughts of death are uncommon in the young, and much more frequent among the elderly. However, HIV and AIDS is associated with death and many adolescents may have to deal with death and grief issues early in their life. As their peers may not have similar challenges their social support and normative informing may be limited and make the experience more difficult.
- Counselling needs – Adolescents may find it difficult to access counselling, especially individual support if they are in a unit where input is focussed at the family. Draimin *et al.*, (1992) noted that although there was overall satisfaction with counselling for those who had received this input, 57% had no counselling in the previous two years. Barriers to counselling access were associated with multiple factors.
- Language – There is some evidence that HIV disease may affect receptive and expressive language in younger children. It is unclear to what extent this continues or exacerbates in adolescents. The language effects may be accounted for by a number of factors, underpinned by documented direct HIV effects on the central nervous system. (Wolters *et al.*, 1995)
- Physical development – Physical development may also be affected. Weight and length is noted below the 50th percentile in children born to HIV infected mothers (Saavedra *et al.*, 1995), although HIV negative children catch up. No follow up into adolescents is available. There is a wide literature in psychology which explores how physical development may interact with psychological and personality development. If there are any physical development obstacles for adolescents with HIV, this literature should be consulted to inform input.

★ Educational needs – Papola *et al.* (1994) note that school age children with HIV may need specific input as they noted deficits in cognitive and learning areas. The services they needed included alternative homes, supplementary education and counselling interventions. Longevity needs to be taken into account. For adolescents, equal school provision and ongoing educational needs are paramount. Cognitive deficits are not universal and many adolescents will face the same educational challenges as other children. Disruption to education is a problem for a person who may have bouts of hospitalisation or who may have frequent hospital appointments.

CARE

The care of underage children is a challenge for all communities where HIV permeates. Care encompasses health and psyshosocial care in the presence of HIV and as a result of bereavement from AIDS. For many adolescents, both these criteria may apply in time. Cohen and Nehring (1994) described foster care for children in a US national study and identified 1,149 HIV positive children in foster care. Policies for foster care of HIV positive children should be carefully thought through and planned in advance. In the Cohen study, 49 states in the USA had specific policies which incorporated training for families, issues of confidentiality, behavioural management, working with natural families, emotional factors, separation and loss, payment, adoption and worries and concerns which may arise. Evans *et al.*, (1994) explored the counselling needs of HIV negative children and adolescents of parents with HIV disease. They noted the repeated hospitalisations which triggered separation for the adolescents which created multiple stressors. The adolescent child is much more likely to be uninfected and may be unidentified in terms of emotional and mental health care. Novel protocols have been set up to provide counselling and care for this needy group.

For many adolescents the tasks of living within an HIV affected family or living beyond an HIV related death are complex. Their burdens are over and above the normal experiences of grief and the ramifications of chronic illness. They may be called on to provide care and nursing for an ill parent and often relied upon to undertake care activities for younger children.

For an adolescent with HIV all this may come at the very point when their own sexuality, their own persona and their own developmental needs are paramount.

AFFECTED YOUTH AND THEIR FAMILY

As the epidemic grows, there will be a number of youth living within a family where at least one person has HIV infection. A family focus allows a more comprehensive understanding and approach to the child, adolescent and adult within the functioning unit (Bor *et al.*, 1993; Wilson, 1993). Niebuhr *et al.* (1994) attempted to enumerate such children as well as explore the perceptions of adults as to their children's emotional needs. Of the 242 patients attending an HIV AIDS clinic, close on a third were parents. Of the female patients, three quarters were mothers and just over a third of these were married. Only half of the parents noted that their children under 4 years of age knew of the diagnosis. Two thirds of the group thought their children had no needs to talk to someone about their parent's health. One in two of the parents felt they did not need any help dealing with their children concerning HIV or AIDS issues.

Siegl and Morse (1994) provided a qualitative study on the experience of parents as they discovered HIV disease in their son. They explored a six stage model which has not been tested out in other groups, but may be helpful in understanding emotional reactions and coping strategies. The six stages were:

Suspecting HIV diseases

Taking in the fact of HIV infection

Going along with the new reality incorporating HIV

Being swept along by symptoms

Beating down the denial reactions

Learning to live with HIV in the family

Roth *et al.*, (1994) set out the wide range of mental health needs resulting from family HIV infections. These authors point out that children in the presence of life threatening illness are at heightened vulnerability for psychological distress. Much of this results from allied separations as well as disruption in nurturing. Emotional well being can be affected by concerns over future loss, disturbed routines and interference with peer relationships as a direct or indirect effect of the illness. These factors can be made more intense by the social stigma and burden of secrecy that may be associated with HIV.

BEREAVEMENT

Many adolescents may be burdened with bereavement, and care for such bereavement is often not forthcoming as needs are unnoticed or unsupported. The effects may be enormous, often with suicidal thoughts or emotional trauma impeding everyday life. Group or individual support for such adolescents is rarely documented (Aronson 1995). The bereaved adolescent may differ markedly from the younger child and from the adult. The issues for younger children may well be concerned with caretaking, concepts of grief and future. The adolescent will have a greater chance of reaching a developmental phase which can cognitively accommodate the notions of death as being permanent and irreversible. However, experience of death may be limited and they have little or no peer group who will provide insight, support or compassion. This may be exacerbated by the fact that the adolescent may need to play a parental role preceding the bereavement which holds the family together but limits the ability of the adolescent to receive attention, support or an independent existence.

The stigma around HIV may also hinder the adolescent in terms of social support or even access to self support sources. For many adolescents bereavements may be multiple and may bring with them emotional and practical burden and strain.

Hudis (1995) identifies four themes that characterise experiences of adolescents who live in families where AIDS is an issue, but they themselves are well. These themes are:

Multiple losses
Isolation and diminished social support
Destructive coping behaviours
Difficulties with new caretaking arrangements

ORPHANS

There is an increasing population of orphans with particularly severe ramifications for adolescents. Foster *et al.*, (1995) enumerated the number of orphans in 570 households in a region of Zimbabwe and noted that by 1992 18.3% include orphans, nearly 12.8% of which were under 15 years of age. Half the deaths since 1987 were as a result of AIDS. This study reported that much of the care was carried out in the extended families, which suffered from strains but exhibited little evidence of discrimination or exploitation of the orphaned children. The emergence of sibling headed orphaned families was noted in this study and may be a challenging problem for the future.

Studies in different centres show different priorities. Levine (1995) elaborated on orphans in the USA and described some of the unmet needs for children, especially around mental health services. Estimates were made in this study based on reported AIDS deaths and these workers predicted that by the end of 1995 maternal death caused by HIV AIDS would have orphaned 24,600 children and 21,000 adolescents in the USA. This pattern would show an upward trend, given that by the end of 1991 13% of US children and 9% of adolescents whose mothers had died of all causes were as a result of AIDS related diseases.

In a study of 541 HIV positive women in the USA across 10 cities, (Schable *et al.*, 1995) 88% had living children, 49% with more than one child. Caretaking patterns were mixed with the most common scenario of a single mother (46) grandparents in 16% of cases and mother and father in only 15%.

In Kinshasa, Ryder *et al.* (1994) studied a longitudinal cohort over a period of four years to track the psychosocial and economic impact of orphans. This sophisticated study compared orphans with an HIV positive mother who was alive and a second control group of children with an HIV negative mother. Of the 1,072 children followed, orphan rates were reported at 8.2 per 100 HIV seropositive women years of follow up. The availability of caring extended family buffeted these growing children against adverse health and socioeconomic effects.

ETHICS AND RIGHTS

Ethical issues are paramount in much of the AIDS debate. The testing ground of any principal usually emerges when the issue is applied to children and adolescents. Ethical challenges emerge in the provision of care, the code of conduct for research, drug treatments, confidentiality, parental involvement and decision making to mention a few. Few issues have been tested out in practice. Three rights of the child are considered in a paper by Oletto *et al.*, (1994) namely right to life, security and socialisation.

A number of factors challenging care in adults, may need explicit consideration and policy when adolescents are involved. This includes areas such as disclosure, informed consent and access to drug trials. Treatment issues may also emerge as ethical and policy questions for this group.

CONCLUSION

It is sad to see the HIV epidemic unfold with such inadequate or inappropriate focus on adolescents. The time has now come to put into practice the findings of the multitude of pen and paper studies on attitudes of youth the world over, and to concentrate the resources on those struggling to live a meaningful life in the presence of HIV.

REFERENCES

Aronson, S. (1995) Five girls in search of a group a group experience for adolescents of parents with AIDS *Int J Group Psychother,* **45**, 223-35.

Bochow, M., Chiarotti, F., Davies, P., *et al.* (1994) Sexual behaviour of a gay and bisexual men in eight European Countries *AIDS Care* vol. 6 no 5, 533-550.

Bor, R. Miller R. and Goldman, E. (1993) HIV AIDS and the family A review of research in the first decade. *Jnl of Family Therapy,* **15**, 187-204.

Bor, R. Miller, R. and Goldman, E. (1992) Theory and Practice of HIV counselling Cassell, London.

Borden, W. (1989) Life review as a therapeutic frame in the treatment of young adults with AIDS *Health and Social work* 14, **4**, 253-259.

Brown, L., Barcone, V., Fritz, G., Cebellero, P., Nassau, J. (1991) AIDS Education The Rhode Island Experience *Health Education Quarterly* **18**, 195-206.

Brown, L., DiClemente, R., Beausoleil, N. (1992) Comparison of HIV related knowledge, attitudes intentions and behaviours among sexually active and abstinent young adolescents *Jnl of Adolescent Health* **13**, 140-145.

Bulterys, M. Chao, A. Habimana, (1994) Incident HIV 1 infection in a cohort of young women in Butare Rwanda. *AIDS* 8, **11**, 1585-1591.

Caselli, D. (1989) Uncommon source for HIV vertical transmission in Italy WHO Paris Conference Abstract B29.

Chen, L.C., Amor, J.S. and Segal, S.J. (1991) AIDS and women's reproductive health, New York: Plenum Press.

Claydon, E., Murphy, S., Osborn, E. *et al* (1991) Rape and HIV *Int J Std AIDS*, **2**, 200-201.

Cohen, F., Nehring, W. (1994) Foster care of HIV positive children in the US Public Health Rep **109**, 60-67.

D'Angelo, L. (1994) HIV infection and AIDS in adolescents in Pediatric AIDS the Challenge of HIV infection in infants children and adolescents 2nd ed. Pizzo, P. and Wilfert, C. Baltimore: Williams and Wilkins.

DiJohn, D. (1990) Paper presented at VI Int Conf on AIDS San Francisco Abstract THC 565.

Durfee (1995) Paper presented at the Japan AIDS Conference Abstract no. PBO443.

Evans, M., Cohen, C., Shidlo, A., De Caprariis, P.P. (1994) Counseling HIV negative children of parents with HIV disease a structured protocol *AIDS Pat Care*, **8**, 16-19.

Forsyth, B. (1995) A pandemic out of control The Epidemiology of AIDS in Geballe, S., Gruendel, J. and Andiman, W. (1995) Forgotten Children of the AIDS Epidemic, New Haven: Yale University Press.

Foster, G., Shakespeare, R., Chinemana, F. (1995) Orphan prevalence and extended family care in a periurban community in Zimbabwe *AIDS Care* **7**, 3-17.

Futterman, D., and Hein, K. (1994) Medical Management of children and adolescents with HIV infection in Pizzo P and Wilfert C (ed) *Pediatric AIDS*, Williams and Wilkins Baltimore 757-772.

Garacia, (1995) Paper presented at the Japan International AIDS Conference Abstract PCO 161.

Gellert, G., Duree M. Berkowitz, C., Higgins, K., Tubiolo, V. (1993) Situational and Sociodemographic characteristics of children infected with HIV from pediatric sexual abuse *Pediatrics* **91**, 39-44.

Gertner, J., Kaufman, F., Donfield, S., Sleeper, L., Shapiro, A., Howard, C. (1994) Delayed somatic growth and pubertal development in HIV infected hemophiliac boys *J Pediatr* **124**, 896-902.

Goldsmith, J. (1994) Medical Management of children and adolescents with Haemophilia in Pizzo P and Wilfert C (ed.) Baltimore: Williams and Wilkins

Goodman, E., Tipton, A., Hecht, L., Chesney, M. (1994) Perserverance pays off health care providers impact on HIV testing decisions by adolescent females *Pediatrics* **94**, 878-82.

Grubman, S., Gross, E., Lerner Weiss, (1995) Older children and adolescents living with perinatally acquired immunodeficiency virus infection *Pediatrics* **95**, 657-663.

Gutman, L.T. (1994) Sexually transmitted diseases in children and adolescents with HIV infection in Pizzo P and Wilfert C (ed.) Pediatric AIDS 2nd ed Baltimore: Williams and Wilkins.

Hein, K., Dell, R., Futterman, D. *et al.* (1995) Comparison of HIV+ and HIV- adolescents risk factors and psychosocial determinants *Pediatrics* **95**, 96-104.

Hooper, S., Whitt, J., Tennison, M. (1993) Behavioural adaptation to HIV seropositive status in children and adolescents with Hemophilia *Am J Dis Child* **147**, 541-545.

Hudis, J. (1995) adolescents living in families with AIDS in Geballe, S. Gruendel, J and Andiman, W. (1995) Forgotten Children of the AIDS Epidemic, New Haven: Yale University Press,

Kaplan M Schonberg S (1994) HIV in adolescents *Clin Perinatol* **21**, 75-84.

Keller, M., (1993) Why dont young adults protect themselves against sexual transmission of HIV? Possible answers to a complex question *AIDS Educ Prev* **5**, 220-233.

Klusman, D. Weber, A., Schmidt, G. (1993) The threat of AIDS perceived by 16 and 17 year old adolescents *AIDS Forschung* **8**, 81-85.

Levy, S., Lampman, C., Handler, A., Play, B., Weeks, K. (1993) Young adolescent attitudes toward sex and substance use implications for AIDS prevention *AIDS Educ Prev* **5**, 340-351.

Lindegren, A. (1995) Paper presented at the Japan International AIDS Conference Abstract no. PC0401.

Konings, E., Blattner, W., Levin, A., Brubaker, G., Siso, Z., Shao, J. (1994) Sexual behaviour survey in a rural area of northwest Tanzania *AIDS* **8**, 99987-99983.

Lemp, G., Hirozawa, A., Givertz, D., Nieri, G., Anderson, L., Lindegrem, M. (1994) Seroprevalence of HIV and risk behaviours among young homosexual and bisexual men The San Francisco Berkeley Young Men's Survey *JAMA* **272**, 449-454.

Levine, C. (1995) Todays Challenges Tomorrow's Dilemmas in Geballe S Gruendel J and Andiman W (eds.) Forgotten children of the AIDS epidemics New Haven: Yale University Press,

Levine, M. (1992) Estimates of the number of motherless youth orphaned by AIDS in the US *JAMA* **268**, 3456-3461.

Lheude, D., Moore, S. (1994) AIDS vulnerability of homeless youth *Venereology* 7, 117-123.

Magura, S. Shapiro, J, Kang, S. (1994) Condom use among criminally involved adolescents *AIDS Care* **6**, 595-603.

Main, D., Iverson, D., McGloin, J. (1994) Comparison of HIV risk behaviours and demographics of adolescents tested or not tested for HIV infection *Public Health Rep* **109**, 699-707.

Maxwell, A., Bastanii, R., Yan, K. (1995) AIDS risk behaviours and correlates in teenagers attending sexually transmitted disease clinics in LA *Genitourin Med* **71**, 82-87.

McCabe, E., Jaffe, L., Diaz, A. (1993) HIV seropositivity in adolescents with syphilis *Pediatrics* **92**, 695-698.

Miller, R. (1995) Guidelines for counselling adolescents with haemophilia and HIV infection and their families *AIDS Care* 7, 381-389.

Moscicki, A., Millestein, S., Broering, J., Irwin, C. (1993) Risks of HIV infection among adolescents attending three diverse clinics *J Pediatr* **122**, 813-820.

Mulder, D., Nunn, A., Kamali, A., (1994) Two Year HIV 1 associated mortality in a Ugandan Rural population *Lancet* **343**, 8904, 1021-1023.

Murphy, S., Kitchen, V., Harris, J., Forster, S. (1989) Rape and subsequent seroconversion to HIV *BMJ* **299**, 718.

Niebuhr, V., Hughes, J., Pollard, R., (1994) Parents with HIV infection perceptions of their children's emotional needs *Pediatr* **93**, 421-426.

Oletto, S., Giaquinto, C., Seefried, M. *et al.* (1994) Paediatric AIDS a new child abuse *Acta Paediatr* **83**, supl. 400, 99-101.

Orr., D., Langeeld, C. (1993) Factors associated with condom use by sexually active male adolescents at risk for *STD Pediatrics*, **91**, 873-879.

Osmond, D., Page, K., Wiley, J. (1994) HIV infection in homosexual and bisexual men 18 to 29 years of age. The San Francisco Young Men's Health Study *Am J Public Health* **84**, 1933-1937.

Papola, P., Alvarez, M., Cohen, H. (1994) Developmental and service needs of school age children with HIV infection a descriptive study *Pediatrics* **94**, 914-918.

Pizzo P and Wilfert C (1994) Pediatric AIDS, The Challenge of HIV infection in infants, children and adolescents, 2nd ed. Baltimore: Williams and Wilkins.

Ponton, L., DiClemente, R., McKenna, S. (1991) An AIDS education and prevention program for hospitalized adolescents. *Journal of the American Academy of Child and*

Adolescent Psychiatry **30** 729-734

Raab, G., Burns, S., Scott, G. (1995) HIV prevalence and risk factors in University students *AIDS* **9**, 191-197.

Ramafedi, G. Lauer, T. (1995) Survival trends in adolescents with HIV infection *Arch Pediatr Adolesc Med* **149**, 1093-1096.

Rawitscher, L., Saitz, R., Friedman, L. (1995) Adolescents preferences regarding HIV related physician counselling and HIV testing *Pediatrics* **96**, 52-58.

Reid, E. (1977) The Lessons of Cairo in Sherr, L. (Ed) AIDS as a Gender Issue, London: Taylor and Francis.

Rosenberg, P. Goedert, J., Biggar, R. (1994) Effect of age at seroconversion on the natural AIDS incubation distribution *AIDS* **8**, 803-810.

Roth, J., Siegel, R., Black, S. (1994) Identifying the mental health needs of children living in families with AIDS or HIV infection *Community Mental Health Journal* 30, 581-593.

Rotheram Borus, M., Reid, H., Rosario, M. (1994) Factors mediating changes in sexual HIV risk behaviour among gay and bisexual male adolescents *Am J Public Health* **84**, 1938-1946.

Ryder, R., Kamenga, M., Nkusu, M., Batter, V., Heyward, W. (1994) AIDS orphans in Kinshasa Zaire Incidence and socioeconomic consequences *AIDS* **8**, 673-679.

Saavedra, J., Henderson, R., Perman, J. *et al.* (1995) Longitudinal assessment of growth in children born to mothers with HIV infection *Arch Pediatr Adolesc Med* **149**, 497-502.

Schable, B. Diaz, T., Chu, S. *et al.* (1995) Who are the primary caretakers of children born to HIV infected mothers. Results from a multistate surveillance project *Pediatrics* **95**, 511-515.

Sellers, D., McGraw, S., KmKinlay, J. (1994) Does the promotion and distribution of condoms increase teen sexual activity? Evidence from an HIV prevention program for Latino Youth *Am J Public Health*, **84**, 12, 1952-1959.

Shaffer, D.R. (1993) Developmental Psychology Brooks Cole (3rd edition) California.

Sherr, L., Hedge, B., Melvin, D., Glover, L., Petrak, J. (1993) Emotional trauma of HIV and AIDS for women *Counsel Psychol Q* **6**, 99.

Sherr, L. (1995) Children and AIDS *AIDS Care Vol.* 7, no.1, 85-89.

Siegl, D., Morse, J. (1994) Tolerating reality the experience of parents of HIV positive sons *Soc Sci Med* **38**, 959-971.

Stevens (1995) Paper presented at the Japan International AIDS Conference Abstract No. PC0420.

Turner, B., Eppes, S., McKee. L., Cosler, L., Mrkon L. (1995) A population based comparison of the clinical course of children and adults with AIDS *AIDS* **9**, 65-72.

Turtle, A. Atshkar, I., Bertuch, M. Dale, M., Hardaker, A. (1994) Reactions to HIV/AIDS of unemployed Australia youth in varying living situations *Venerology*, 7, 125-129.

Van den berg, H., Gerritsen, E. Van Tol, M., Dooren, L., Vossen, J. (1994) Ten years after acquiring an HIV 1 infection – a study in a cohort of eleven neonates infected by aliquots from a single plasma donation *Acta Paediatr* **83**, 173-178.

Wilson, P. (1993) HIV disease toward comprehensive services for families in Lynch, V., Lloyd, G., and Fimbres, M. Eds. The changing face of AIDS Implications for social work practice, Westport: Auburn House.

Wolters, P., Brouwers, P., Moss H., Pizzo, P. (1995) Differential receptive and expressive language functioning of children with symptomatic HIV disease and relation to CT scan brain abnormalities *Pediatrics* **95**, p. 112-119.

3

HIV and AIDS in Adolescence: Epidemiology

JONATHAN ELFORD

Adolescence may be seen as a transitional period in human development - from being a child to an adult, from minor to major, from dependency to responsibility... from HIV to AIDS. With its prolonged incubation period of ten years or more (Munoz *et al.*, 1989), most of those infected with HIV during adolescence will only develop AIDS after they have left their teenage years behind them. Consequently, most people diagnosed with AIDS in their twenties would almost certainly have been infected with HIV during their adolescence.

For this reason any epidemiological investigation of HIV infection acquired in adolescence must consider AIDS among people in their twenties. Similarly, AIDS and severe HIV disease seen in adolescents may reflect HIV infection that actually occurred in childhood. While paediatric HIV infection falls outside the remit of this chapter, its intimate relationship with AIDS in adolescence must be borne in mind.

This chapter first considers HIV and AIDS surveillance data from Europe, the United Kingdom alone and the United States of America and then reviews information gathered in HIV seroprevalence and incidence surveys from around the world.

HIV AND AIDS SURVEILLANCE

Summary Interpretation of HIV and AIDS surveillance data can be problematic since the true population at risk is often unknown and rates cannot be reliably estimated. Nonetheless, patterns of infection among people with HIV or AIDS can be revealing despite the absence of a denominator.

The key epidemiological features of HIV and AIDS in adolescence as revealed through European and US surveillance data were:

- Females with AIDS were more likely to have been infected during adolescence than males.
- Sex between men accounted for most cases of sexually acquired HIV infection among adolescent males.
- Females outnumbered males among adolescents with heterosexually-acquired HIV infection.
- In Europe, about half the injecting drug users with AIDS were infected with HIV in adolescence.
- The risk of HIV infection increased steadily with age during adolescence and into the twenties.

Europe, AIDS surveillance

Nearly 130,000 cases of AIDS had been reported by 44 European countries at the end of September 1994 (European Centre for the Epidemiological Monitoring of AIDS, 1994). Of these, 854 – less than 1% - were diagnosed in adolescents aged 13-19 years. A further 36,769 cases – nearly 30% of the total – were reported among young adults aged 20-29 years, many of whom would have been infected with HIV during adolescence (Table 1). While epidemiological patterns vary from one European country to another, it is nonetheless useful to consider Europe as a whole before examining data for the UK alone.

In Europe, a far higher proportion of females with AIDS appear to have been infected with HIV in adolescence than males. Forty percent of all females with AIDS were diagnosed in their twenties compared with 27% of males (Table 1). HIV infection most probably occurred during adolescence for both males and females alike since rates of progression from seroconversion to AIDS are believed to be similar for both sexes (Melnick *et al.* 1994)

Exposure category

13-19 years The transfusion of blood or blood products for coagulation disorders, in particular haemophilia, accounted for most AIDS diagnosis (61%) among adolescents males (Figure 1)[1]. In many cases, transfusion and infection with HIV would have occurred in childhood. With the introduction of heat treatment

[1]Only HIV and AIDS cases with a reported exposure category are included in figures 1, 2, 4 - 7. The excluded "other/undetermined" category accounted for 0.3 - 4.8% of AIDS and HIV diagnosis in the UK (depending on the age group) and 2.0 - 10.6% of AIDS cases reported in all Europe.

Table 1
Europe, AIDS cases reported by 30 September 1994

Age group (years)	Males No.	Males %	Females No.	Females %	Total No.	Total %
0 - 12	2,699	(2.5)	2,105	(9.9)	4,804	(3.8)
13 - 19	684	(0.6)	170	(0.8)	854	(0.7)
20 - 24	5,584	(5.3)	2,244	(10.5)	7,828	(6.1)
25 - 29	22,554	(21.3)	6,387	(29.9)	28,941	(22.7)
≥ 30	74,156	(70.0)	10,369	(48.6)	84,525	(66.4)
TOTAL*	105,978	(100.0)	21,343	(100.0)	127,321	(100.0)

*includes 301 males and 68 females of unknown age

of blood products and the screening of donated blood since the 1980s, the risk associated with this particular exposure has virtually fallen to zero. Consequently, this exposure category will account for a diminishing proportion of AIDS cases over time.

Among adolescent males with AIDS whose exposure to HIV was *behaviour-related,* injecting drug use accounted for a greater proportion of cases (24%) than sexual intercourse (14%) (Figure 1). A similar pattern was seen in adolescent

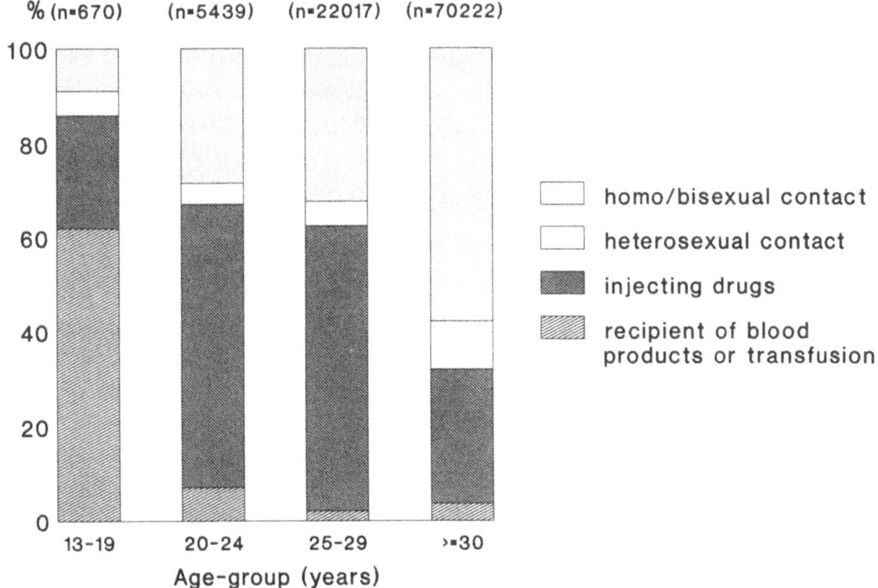

Fig. 1 AIDS cases reported among males in Europe to 30 September 1994 by exposure category

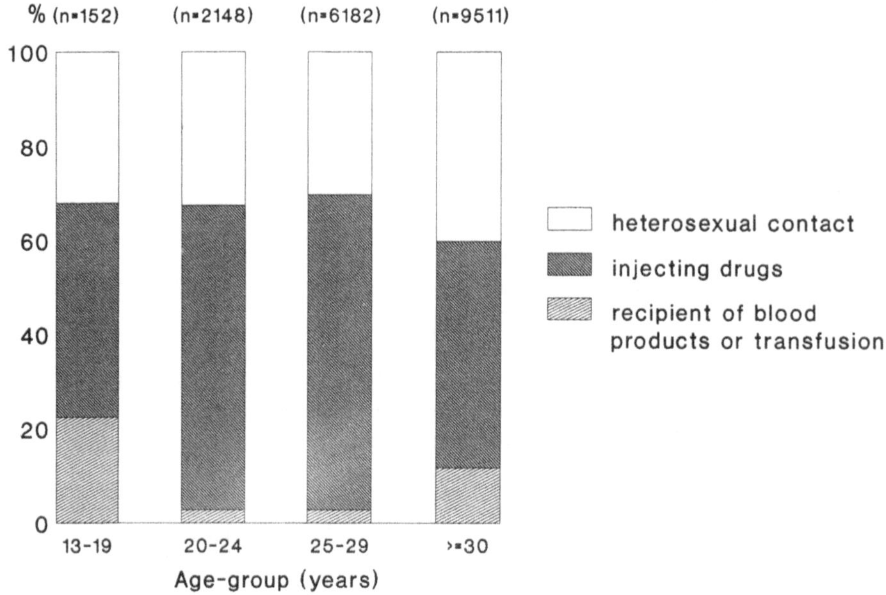

Fig. 2 AIDS cases reported among females in Europe to 30 September 1994 by exposure category

females with more than 40% of AIDS cases being associated with injecting drug use (Figure 2). Among adolescent males with AIDS whose exposure category was sexual intercourse, however, more reported having had sex with another man (9%) than with a female partner alone (6%) (Figure 1).

20-29 years Behaviour-related exposures accounted for the vast majority of cases among young adults diagnosed with AIDS in their twenties (and probably infected with HIV in adolescence). In this age group injecting drug use also accounted for a far higher proportion of cases than sexual contact (Figures 1 and 2). Twice as many females aged 20-29 years reported injecting drug use (64%) rather than sexual contact (30%) as their exposure category (males 59% and 36% respectively).

Homosexual contact Men diagnosed with AIDS in their twenties who acquired HIV through sexual contact were more likely to report having had sex with another man (31%) than with a woman alone (5%) (Figure 1). Of those young men who acquired HIV through sexual contact, the percentage reporting homo/bisexual contact steadily declined from 93% (240/258) in 1985 to 81% (1,036/1,276) in 1993. If this trend continues, an increasing proportion of AIDS cases will be seen in young men who report having sex with women rather than men. Despite this shift, for the foreseeable future adolescents males who have sex with other men will continue to account for most cases of sexually acquired HIV infection among teenage boys.

Heterosexual contact Women outnumbered men by about 2 to 1 (2,583 females, 1,396 males) among those who were diagnosed with AIDS in their twenties reporting heterosexual contact. In many cases, infection would have occurred during adolescence. This pattern was reversed above the age of 30 years; 7,169 males and 3,826 females reported heterosexual contact as their exposure category. Consequently, among people with AIDS reporting heterosexual contact, 40% of females but only 10% of males were diagnosed in their twenties (and probably infected with HIV as teenagers). It appears that where the risk for HIV was heterosexual contact females were more likely to have been infected in adolescence than males.

How can this excess of young females acquiring HIV through heterosexual contact in adolescence be explained? A partial explanation is that females are more likely than males to report having had heterosexual contact with high risk partners such as injecting drug users (PHLS, Communicable Disease Surveillance Centre, 1995). But other factors need to considered. For example, are adolescent females more likely to have sexual relations with older men? Are young women more susceptible to HIV infection for physiological reasons? Are they more likely to have cofactors such as undiagnosed sexually transmissible diseases? Clearly the differential seen in the number of females and males who appear to have acquired HIV infection through heterosexual contact in adolescence needs further examination.

Drugs Overall, approximately one quarter of males and 40% of all females with AIDS were diagnosed in their twenties (and probably infected with HIV in adolescence) (Table 1). These proportions varied between exposure categories, however. Among male injecting drug users with AIDS, 45% (16,545/36,690) were diagnosed in their twenties, while for females the corresponding figure was 54% (5,524/10,222). It appears that about half the people with AIDS who acquired their infection through injecting drugs were infected with HIV in adolescence, as a result of needle sharing. In no other exposure category was the proportion seemingly infected in adolescence so high.

Age and time trends

The number of people diagnosed with AIDS increases steadily with age among adolescents and people in their twenties (Figure 3). (Data on individual age were only available for ten European countries, 4,949 AIDS cases). There were 1127 AIDS diagnosis in males and females aged 23-25 years compared with 2,619 in those aged 27-29 years. AIDS diagnosed in people in their twenties generally reflects HIV infection that occurred an average of ten years earlier, when they were teenagers. Assuming similar rates of progression across this age group, these data are consistent with the risk of HIV infection increasing steadily with age throughout adolescence. This is not altogether surprising. Adolescence marks a period of rapid development and experimentation – with sex and drugs – which increases with age.

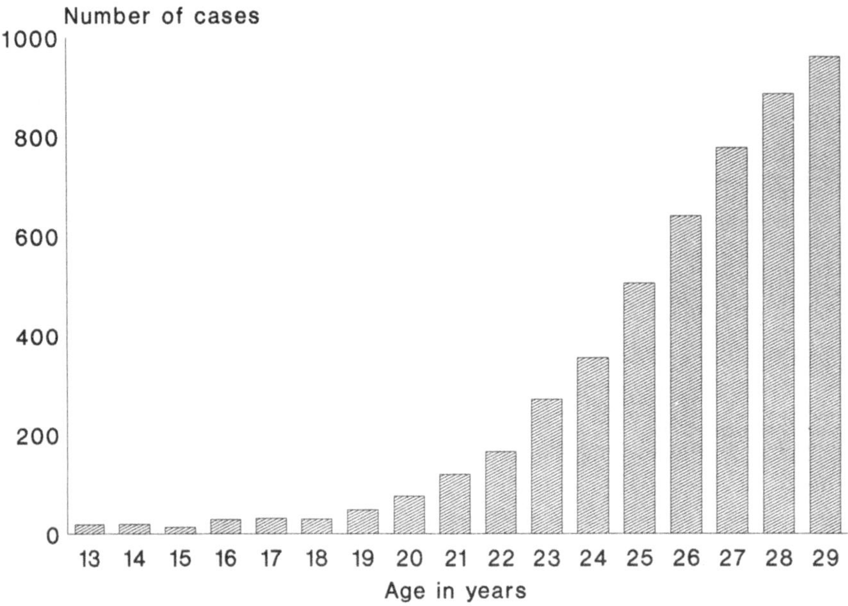

Fig. 3 AIDS cases reported in Europe to 30 September 1994 by age at diagnosis

Among females aged 25-29 years at AIDS diagnosis, there has been a steady and sustained rise in the annual number of cases in all exposure categories through to 1993 (1994 was excluded because of possible reporting delay). A similar pattern was seen in males of the same age except for men infected through blood and blood products whose numbers declined in 1992 and 1993.

The sustained annual increase in the number of AIDS diagnosis, continuing into the 1990s among people aged 25-29 years reflects in part a corresponding annual increase in exposure to HIV among adolescents in the early 1980s. That teenagers have continued to face an increasing risk of HIV infection into the 1990s is revealed through HIV surveillance and seroprevalence/incidence studies, considered later in the chapter.

United Kingdom, AIDS surveillance

In the United Kingdom, just over 10,000 cases of AIDS had been reported by 31 December 1994 (PHLS Communicable Disease Surveillance Centre, 1995). Of these, 68 – less than 1% of the total – were diagnosed in adolescents aged 13-19 years, a similar proportion to all Europe. A further 2,179 cases (21% of the total) were diagnosed in young adults aged 20-29 years, many of whom would have been infected with HIV in adolescence (Table 2). This percentage was less than that for all Europe where 30% of people with AIDS were diagnosed in their twenties.

Table 2
United Kingdom, AIDS cases reported by 31 December 1994

Age group (years)	Males No.	%	Females No.	%	Total No.	%
0 - 12	90	(1.0)	86	(9.7)	176	(1.7)
13 - 19	59	(0.6)	9	(1.0)	68	(0.7)
20 - 24	348	(3.7)	98	(11.0)	446	(4.3)
25 - 29	1,484	(15.8)	249	(28.0)	1,733	(16.8)
≥ 30	7,403	(78.6)	446	(50.1)	7,849	(76.2)
TOTAL*	9,414	(100.0)	890	(100.0)	10,304	(100.0)

*includes 30 males and 2 femals of unknown age

In many respects the epidemiological characteristics of AIDS among adolescents and young adults seen in the UK reflect those seen in all Europe. For example, a greater proportion of females with AIDS were diagnosed in their teens of twenties than males (40 v 20%) (Table 2). Transfusion of blood and blood products accounted for the overwhelming majority of AIDS cases diagnosed in adolescent males (Figure 4), although most of these (200/228; 88%) were diagnosed before 1987. The heat treatment of blood products and screening of donated blood since

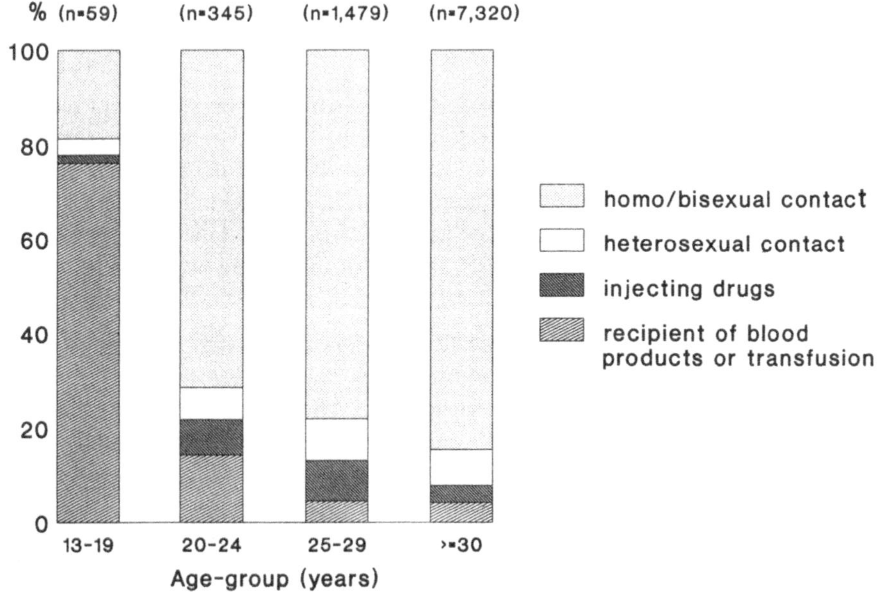

Fig. 4 AIDS cases reported among males in the United Kingdom to 31 December 1994 by exposure category

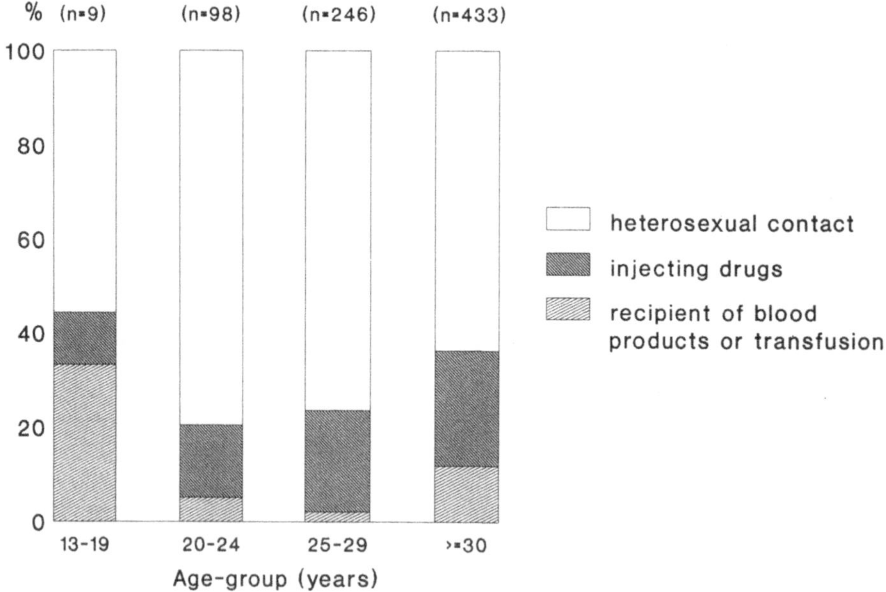

Fig. 5 AIDS cases reported among females in the United Kingdom to 31 December 1994 by exposure category

the mid 1980s have virtually reduced the risk of HIV transmission associated with this exposure category to zero.

Males diagnosed with AIDS as teenagers or in their twenties who acquired HIV through sexual contact were more likely to have had sex with another man than with a woman (Figure 4). Among those reporting sexual contact as their risk, the percentage who had sex with another man declined 97% to 83% between 1985 and 1993. A similar decline was seen in all Europe. Despite this fall, sex between men continued to account for most AIDS cases among young men with sexually acquired HIV infection.

Females outnumbered males by 2 to 1 (271 v 155) among people diagnosed with AIDS aged 13-29 years reporting heterosexual contact. Over the age of 30 this pattern was reversed, a pattern seen in all Europe. The number of AIDS diagnoses increased steadily with age between 20 and 29 years, reflecting an equally steady increase in the risk of acquiring HIV infection during adolescence when infection is likely to have occurred.

What then were the epidemiological differences between all Europe and the United Kingdom? The most striking difference concerned the proportion of AIDS cases attributed to injecting drug use and sexual contact. In all Europe, adolescents and young adults with AIDS reporting a behaviour-related exposure were more likely to report injecting drug use rather than sexual contact as their risk (Figures 1 and 2). The reverse was the case in the UK (Figures 4 and 5). For males diagnosed with AIDS between 13 and 29 years, 1,568 reported sexual contact as their risk, compared with 154 whose risk was injecting drugs. For females the corresponding figures were 271 and 69. This difference between the all Europe and UK data reflects the well established fact that in the UK, HIV prevalence and incidence among injecting drug users is lower than that reported in gay men (Noone *et al.*, 1993; CDSC, 1995). In many European countries, on the other hand, injecting drug use presents a greater risk for HIV than sex between men.

United Kingdom, HIV surveillance

Surveillance of newly diagnosed HIV infection provides information on more recent infection than AIDS surveillance data, which reflect patterns prevailing an average of ten years before AIDS diagnosis. Information is rarely available on when HIV infection occurred, however, except for those people with a previous negative test result. Consequently HIV surveillance data are only available for the year and age when the person received the positive test result rather than year and age of infection. Some people who were in their twenties when they first tested positive for HIV antibody may have been infected during adolescence, although this is less clear cut than with an AIDS diagnosis. Similarly, some of those who tested positive between 13-19 years of age will have been infected before adolescence. For the purposes of this analysis I have assumed that the majority of those aged 20-24 years when they tested positive for HIV antibody were infected in adolescence. A further limitation of HIV surveillance is that differential patterns of HIV infection by age or exposure category may, in part, reflect corresponding differentials in the propensity to seek an HIV test rather than true differences in the risk of infection. Despite these caveats, HIV surveillance data provide an important complement to the information gathered through AIDS surveillance.

In the United Kingdom 23,063 people had been diagnosed with HIV infection (19,862 males, 3,201 females) by 31 December 1994 (PHLS Communicable Disease Surveillance Center, 1995). There is a remarkable consistency between the epidemiological patterns described by both HIV and AIDS surveillance data among adolescents and young adults in the United Kingdom. This suggests that patterns of HIV infection which prevailed in the early to mid 1980s (as reflected in AIDS surveillance data) have persisted into the 1990s.

Only 3% of all HIV infections were reported among adolescents, but a further 15% were reported in 20-24 year olds (Table 3). A greater proportion of females with HIV infection appear to have been infected in adolescence than males. Of the females with HIV infection, 30% were aged 13-24 years at diagnosis compared with 17% of the males (Table 3). A similar pattern was seen for AIDS diagnoses (Table 2).

Most adolescent males with HIV were infected as a result of the transfusion of blood or blood products although this percentage has decreased steadily over time. Among adolescent males with a behaviour-related exposure, sexual contact with

Table 3
United Kingdom, HIV diagnoses reported by 31 December 1994

Age group (years)	Males No.	Males %	Females No.	Females %	Total No.	Total %
0 - 12	340	(1.7)	155	(4.8)	495	(2.1)
13 - 19	588	(3.0)	146	(4.6)	734	(3.2)
20 - 24	2,711	(13.6)	808	(25.2)	3,519	(15.3)
25 - 29	4,598	(23.1)	955	(29.8)	5,553	(24.1)
≥ 30	11,252	(56.7)	1,076	(33.6)	12,328	(53.5)
TOTAL*	19,862	(100.0)	3,201	(100.0)	23,063	(100.0)

*includes 373 males and 61 females of unkown age

another male was the most common risk for HIV infection. Injecting drug use, however, accounted for a larger proportion of reported HIV infections among adolescents and people in their early twenties (Figures 6 and 7) than was seen for AIDS (Figures 4 and 5). Indeed, among adolescent females, injecting drug use and heterosexual contact accounted for an equal number of HIV infections raising the possibility that injecting drug use has presented an increasing risk for HIV infection among teenagers in recent years. The availability of HIV testing facilities for drug users attending clinics could, however, have confounded this pattern.

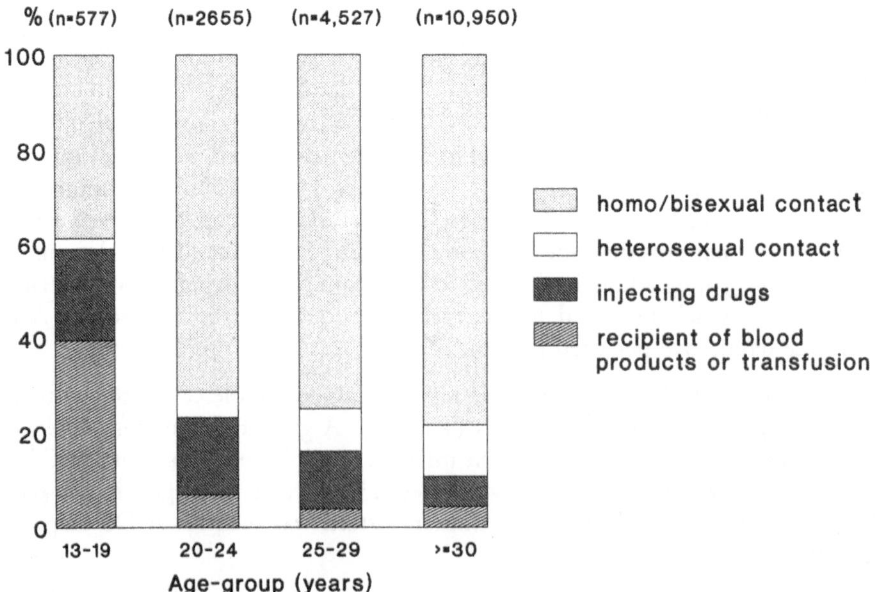

Fig. 6 HIV diagnoses reported among males in the United Kingdom to 31 December 1994 by exposure category

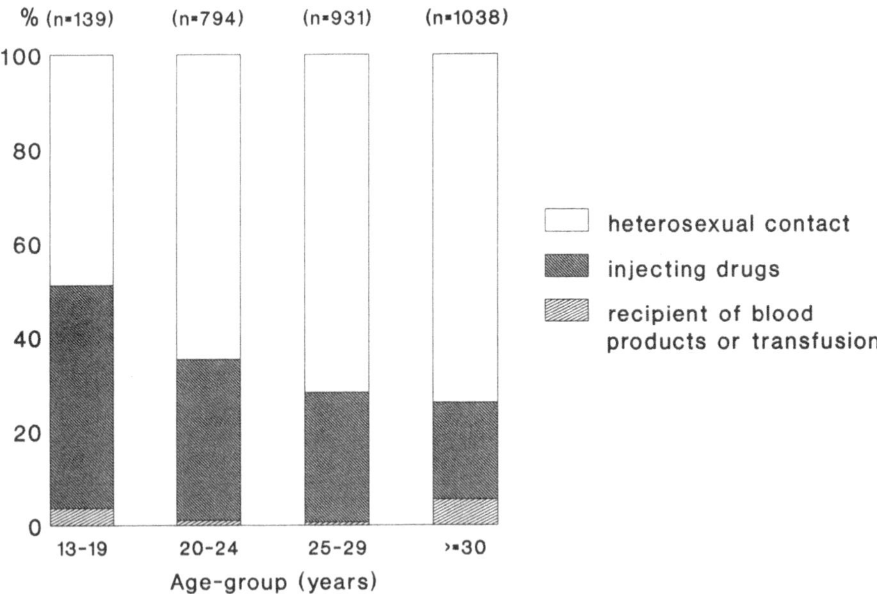

Fig. 7 HIV diagnoses reported among females in the United Kingdom to 31 December 1994 by exposure category

Among males aged 13-24 years with sexually-acquired HIV infection, there was a steady decline in the percentage who reported sex with another man from 100% in 1985 to 90% in 1993. A similar decline was seen for AIDS diagnoses. Nonetheless, HIV surveillance data for 1993 confirm that for adolescent males, sex with another man continues to present a greater risk for HIV infection than sex with a woman.

United States of America, AIDS surveillance

The epidemiological characteristics of AIDS among adolescents and young adults in the USA have already been described in detail elsewhere and will not be reproduced here (D'Angelo, 1994; Bowler *et al.*, 1992; Friedman & Goodman, 1992; Gayle and D'Angelo, 1991). In many respects they reflect the patterns seen in the UK rather than in all Europe. In brief, among adolescent males with AIDS the transfusion of blood and blood products accounted for nearly half the cases reported through to June 1994 (CDC, 1994). But for adolescent males with AIDS whose risk was behaviour-related, sexual contact particularly with men accounted for far more cases than injecting drug use. Likewise, more adolescent females with AIDS reported sexual contact as their exposure category rather than injecting drug use. Females outnumbered males by more than 10 to 1 among adolescents with AIDS reporting heterosexual contact – a differential even greater than that reported in the United Kingdom or all Europe.

Sexual contact rather than injecting drug use also accounted for the majority of AIDS cases among males and females diagnosed in their early twenties. Furthermore, three-quarters of men aged 20-24 years reported sex with another man as their risk, while only 3% reported heterosexual contact – a more than 20-fold difference. Again this differential is even greater than that reported in the UK or all Europe.

One of the striking epidemiological features of AIDS in the USA, however, was the disproportionate number of AIDS cases reported among blacks and Hispanics. This is seen in people of all ages, including adolescents and those in their twenties. Approximately 75% of females diagnosed with AIDS in their adolescence or early twenties were black or Hispanic – a figure far in excess of the size of those communities. Half the males diagnosed with AIDS at the same age were either black or Hispanic (Figure 8). Overall black or Hispanic males were more likely than white males to have acquired HIV infection through injecting drug use, although sex between man presented a major risk for all ethnic groups.

HIV SEROPREVALENCE AND INCIDENCE SURVEYS

HIV seroprevalence and incidence surveys provide greater insight into *current* HIV infection among adolescents than AIDS surveillance data. While many epidemiological studies were not specifically designed to examine HIV in adolescence, they nonetheless included younger subjects although the age range

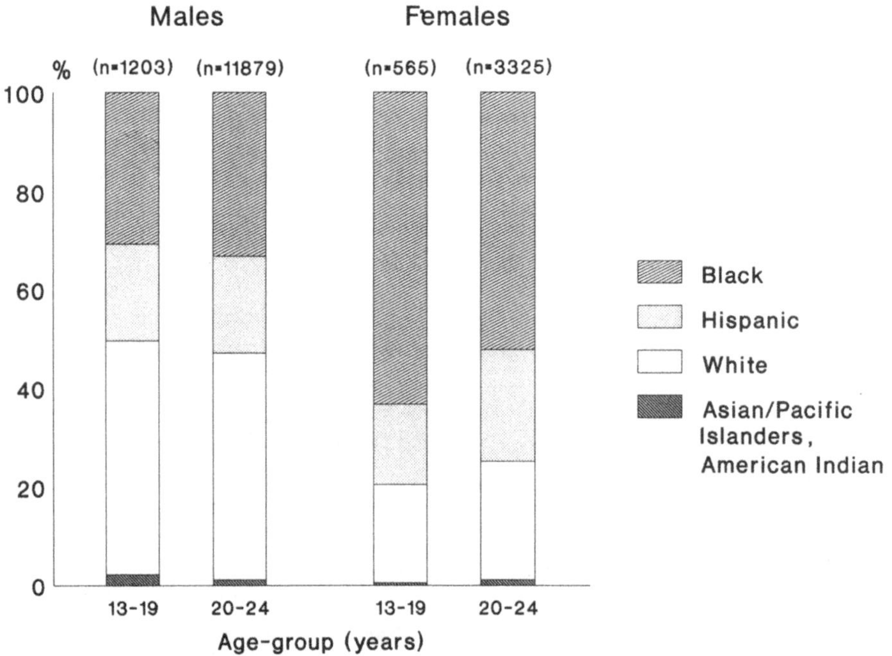

Fig. 8 AIDS cases reported in the United States of America to June 1994 by ethnic group

varied between studies. The most comprehensive epidemiological studies of HIV among adolescents have been conducted in the USA and Africa.

United States of America

Summary Epidemiological studies in the USA generally found that male and female adolescents had similar HIV seroprevalence in marked contrast to the elevated rate seen in men at older ages. In some studies seroprevalence in adolescent females exceeded that in males. Heterosexual contact, male homosexual contact and injecting drug use in adolescence were the major risk factors for HIV infection. HIV seroprevalence increased with age during adolescence and through the twenties but varied widely according to the population studied. Blacks, Hispanics, the economically-disadvantaged and the homeless had the highest seroprevalence and incidence rates at this age.

Seroprevalence / incidence surveys conducted in medical settings

Military applicants All applicants for US military service are tested for HIV antibody during medical screening. Between 1985-89, more than one million teenage applicants aged 17-19 years were tested and 393 (0.34 per 1,000) were found to be HIV positive – males 0.35, females, 0.32 per 1,000. Even in this narrow age band, seroprevalence increased with each year of age and continued to

Table 4
United States of America, HIV seroprevalence surveys conducted in non-medical settings

Population Surveyed	Year	Age group (years)	Sex	Seroprevalence per 1000 (number HIV positive /number tested)		Reference
Military applicants	1985-1989	17-19	M F	0.35 0.32	(345/991,455) (48/150, 043)	Burke et al 1990
Army reserves	1986-1989	17-19	M+F	0.3	(14/46,776)	Cowan et al 1994
College students	1988-1989	18-24	M+F	0.8	(11/13,135)	Gayle et al 1990
Job Corps	1987-1990	16-21	M F	3.7 3.2	(357/96,029) (131/41,168)	St Louis et al 1991
Homeless youth *(San Francisco, New York City, Houston)*	1989-1992	15-24	M F	48.8 13.0	(143/2,926) (40/3,086)	Allen et al 1994
Homeless youth *(New York City)*	1987-1989	15-20	M F	60.2 42.4	(97/1,611) (44/1,037)	Stricof et al 1991

rise among applicants in their twenties. Black teenage applicants had a significantly higher seroprevalence rate than white (1.0 v 0.2 per 1,000). During the study period, annual seroprevalence rates decreased in male applicants (more so for whites than blacks) but increased in black female applicants (there were too few white applicants to examine time trends in this group) (Burke *et al.*, 1990). The exclusion of drug users, and at the time of the survey, homosexuals from the US military service limits the applicability of these findings to a wider population.

Soldiers on active duty are retested for HIV antibody at least every 2 years. Between 1985-89, 718,780 soldiers were tested and 429 seroconversions were detected (HIV seroconversion rate 0.4/1,000 person years). Although overall seroconversion rates declined during the study from 0.5 (1985-87) to 0.3 (1988-1989) per 1,000 person years, seroincidence among black male teenage soldiers more than doubled in that time. The exclusion of drug users and homosexuals again limits the extent to which these findings can be generalised (McNeil, 1991).

US Army Reserve Components US Army Reserve Components comprise people who usually work full time in civilian and part time in military occupations. A seroprevalence of 0.3/1,000 was reported among teenagers aged 17-19 years recruited between 1985-89. In multivariate analysis, males had significantly higher seroprevalence than females, and regardless of age or sex, blacks and Hispanics had 4-5 times the prevalence of whites. Overall, seroprevalence was lowest among teenagers and highest in people in their twenties (Cowan *et al.*, 1994). The same exclusions applied to the Reserve Components as to the military which may limit the applicability of these findings to a broader population.

College Students In a 1988-89 unlinked anonymous survey among students from 19 universities (17 public, 2 private), HIV seroprevalence among 18-24 years olds was 0.8 per 1000 (11/13,135). This rate was higher than that seen in teenage military applicants, partially explained by the exclusion from the armed forces of injecting drug users and (officially) gay men. HIV seroprevalence in college students over the age of 25 years was significantly higher than in the under-25s. Although for the study population as a whole (age range 13-73, median 21) seroprevalence was higher for men than women, sex differences for those aged 18-24 years were not presented in the paper (Gayle *et al.*, 1990).

Job Corps Among 16-21 year olds entering the Job Corps, a federally funded education programme for disadvantaged youth, between 1987-1990 3.6 per 1,000 (488/137,209) were HIV positive – a seroprevalence rate ten times that seen in teenage military applicants. Females aged 16-18 years had higher seroprevalence than males but above this age male rates exceeded females'. Blacks (5.3/1,000) and Hispanics (2.6/1,000) had higher seroprevalence than whites (1.2/1,000). HIV seroprevalence rates increased steadily with each year of age, more so for blacks and Hispanics than whites. While those who actively used drugs were excluded from the Job Corps, homosexuality and a history of drug use did not influence selection. Thus this group was less restricted than military applicants (St Louis *et al.*, 1991)

A subsequent survey among Job Corps entrants revealed increasing seroprevalence between 1988 and 1992 in females, but not males. Consequently, by 1992 female seroprevalence exceeded the male rate. Among black females aged 16-21 years seroprevalence more than doubled between 1988 (3.2/1,000) and 1992 (6.6/1,000) (Conway *et al.*, 1993).

Homeless youth Between 1989-92, an unlinked anonymous HIV seroprevalence survey was conducted among runaway youths aged 15-24 years in hostels for the homeless in San Francisco (2 sites), New York City, Houston and Dallas. Nearly 80% of the subjects were under 20 years old. Of the 2926 males tested, 143 (4.9%) were HIV positive – a seroprevalence rate more than 100 times that seen among male teenage military applicants. Seroprevalence in the five hostels ranged from 0% (Dallas) to 10% (San Francisco). Of the 3086 females, 40 (1.3%) were HIV positive (range 0, Dallas to 2.66% San Francisco). Median seroprevalence for homo/bisexual men was 32.2% compared with 0.8% for heterosexual men. After controlling for age, sex and sexual orientation, median HIV seroprevalence rates were significantly higher among black youths than white at two of the sites (Allen *et al.*, 1994).

In an unlinked anonymous seroprevalence survey among 15-20 year olds attending Covenant House, New York (a facility for runaway and homeless youth) between 1987-1989, 5.3% (142/2,667) were found to be HIV positive. Seroprevalence rates were strongly associated with age, increasing from 1.3% in 15 year olds to 8.6% in 20 year olds. More than a quarter of the males reporting homo/bisexual contact were HIV positive. In multivariate analysis, HIV infection in male adolescents was associated with homo/bisexual activity, prostitution, having had an STD and crack use. For females, the association between HIV infection, prostitution and history of STD were of borderline significance (Stricof *et al.*, 1991).

Seroprevalence / incidence surveys conducted in medical settings

Adolescent medical centre Between 1987-89 an unlinked anonymous seroprevalence survey was conducted among adolescents aged 13-19 years attending the Children's National Medical Center, Washington DC. Nearly 90% of the patients were black. Of the 3520 teenagers surveyed, 13 (3.7 per 1,000) were HIV positive. Seroprevalence was higher in females than males (4.7 v 1.7 per 1,000) and was higher in those aged 15 years and above (4.9 per 1,000) than those under 15 (1.7 per 1,000). All the HIV positive adolescents lived within the Washington city boundaries. A programme of voluntary HIV testing offered to "high risk" individuals attending the clinic between 1987-89 only identified 5 of the 13 patients (38%) detected by the unlinked survey, giving some indication of the degree of undiagnosed HIV in teenagers (D'Angelo *et al.*, 1991).

The first 50 HIV positive adolescents (33 males, 17 females) aged 13-21 years seen by the Adolescent AIDS Program, New York City, were compared with 43 HIV negative adolescents who had been referred to the clinic for testing. Compared with HIV negative controls, HIV positive males were more likely to report anal intercourse with another man and a history of sexual abuse. No other significant differences in risk behaviours were found between the HIV positive and negative adolescents. Nearly half (24) the HIV positive patients had CD4 counts less than 500/mm^3 when they were referred to the program (Futterman *et al.*, 1993)

Table 5
United States of America, HIV seroprevalence surveys conducted in medical facilities

Population Surveyed	Year	Age group (years)	Sex	Seroprevalence per 1000 (number HIV positive /number tested)	Reference
Adolescent medical centre *(Washington DC)*	1987-1989	13-19	M F	1.7 (2/1,175) 4.7 (11/2,345)	D'Angelo et al 1991
HIV testing sites	1991	13-19	M+F	5.0 (1,242/261,942)	CDC 1992
Sentinel hospitals	1988-1989	15-24	M F	10 (data not published) 2 (data not published)	St Louis et al 1990
STD Clinics *(Baltimore)*	1987	15-19	M F	25.3 (11/434) 19.6 (10/509)	Quinn et al 1988
STD Clinics	1988-1989	15-19	M+F	4 (range 0-47) (data not published)	Wendell et al 1992
Neonates	1987-1988	<20*			
New York City			F	7.2 (93/12,871)	Novick et al
Upstate New York			F	1.3 (16/12,344)	1989
Pregnant women *(Atlanta)*	1987-1990	16-20	F	4.0 (31/7,702)	Lindsay et al 1991

*mother's age

HIV testing sites In 1991, HIV counselling and testing services in the USA performed over 2 million antibody tests. Because some clients were tested more than once,. the exact number of persons was unknown. Among adolescents aged 13-19 years, 261,942 tests were performed; of these 1,242 (5 per 1,000) were positive. No further information was provided on the characteristics of adolescents tested for HIV but, overall, seropositivity was highest among Hispanics, blacks, drug users and men who had sex with men (MMWR 1992). This study was based on people who voluntarily sought an HIV test. A national investigation into HIV antibody testing estimated that only 30% of males and approximately one quarter of females aged 18-24 years had ever been tested for HIV (Berrios *et al.,* 1993).

Sentinel hospitals In 1988-89, 26 sentinel hospitals in 21 cities provided blood specimens from inpatients and outpatients for an unlinked anonymous seroprevalence survey. Specimens were excluded if the patient had a diagnosis of AIDS, HIV, any associated conditions or risk factors for HIV. Median seroprevalence at age 15-24 years was 10 per 1,000 per males and 2 per 1,000 for females. In the two hospitals with the highest overall seroprevalence, HIV seroprevalence among 15-19 years olds was 11 per 1,000 (Newark) and 38 per 1,000 (South Bronx) (St Louis *et al.,* 1992)

STD clinic attenders In a 1987 unlinked anonymous survey among people attending STD clinics run by the City Health Department in Baltimore, HIV seroprevalence was 25 per 1,000 in males aged 15-19 years and 20 per 1000 among females. While male and female seroprevalence rates were similar for adolescents and people in their early twenties, over the age of 25 years the male rate was 3 times that seen in females. Multivariate analysis revealed that for males of all ages, including adolescence, HIV infection was associated with black race, homo/bisexual activity, injecting drug use and history of syphilis. For women, including adolescents, injecting drug use and being the sex partner of a drug user was associated with HIV infection. One third of men with HIV, including adolescents, did not acknowledge any risk factors for HIV and two thirds of infected women under 25 years did not do so either (Quinn *et al.*, 1988).

A further study in the same STD clinics in Baltimore retrospectively tested stored sera collected between 1979-83. Combining these data with those collected in 1987-89, the authors examined time trends in HIV seroprevalence between 1979-89. During this period, seroprevalence increased significantly in all age groups, particularly among teenagers whose seroprevalence increased more than ten-fold from 1.8 per 1000 in 1979-83 (5/2,704) to 21 per 1,000 in 1987-89 (36/1,482) ($p<0.001$) (Quinn *et al.*, 1992).

In 1988-89, the Centres for Disease Control conducted a blinded seroprevalence survey in 84 STD clinics in 38 metropolitan areas throughout the USA. Median seroprevalence among 15-19 years olds was 4 per 1,000 (range 0 - 47) rising to 14 per 1,000 (range 0 - 118) in 20-24 year olds. Among 15-19 year old heterosexuals who reported no other risk for HIV (more than 80% of the study population), female seroprevalence rates were higher than males'. Two clinics in Florida reported rates of 83 and 59 per 1,000 in female adolescents reporting heterosexual contact is their sole risk. Teenage boys who had sex with other men had the highest seroprevalence (160 per 1,000) among adolescents. At age 20-24 years, median seroprevalence among men who had sex with men rose to 301 per 1,000 (range 97-558) (Wendell *et al.*, 1992)

Neonates and pregnant women In a 1987-88 unlinked anonymous survey among newborns, HIV seroprevalence in New York City was 7.2 per 1,000 (93/12,871) among infants born to mothers under the age of 20 years compared with 1.3 per 1,000 in the same age group in upstate New York. In both areas, seroprevalence rates were highest in newborns whose mothers were black or Hispanic compared with whites (New York City seroprevalence rates 8.1, 7.7, 1.7 per 1,000 respectively; upstate New York 2.8, 4.0 0.5) Novick *et al.*, 1989).

Between 1987-90, 95% of pregnant women attending Grady Memorial Hospital, Atlanta accepted voluntary HIV testing as part of their antenatal care. Of the 7702 females aged 16-20 years, 31 (4 per 1,000) were positive and 2 of 1,107 females under the age of 16 years (2 per 1,000) tested positive. Seropositive women identified prior to pregnancy were not included in the analysis. Nearly half the young women diagnosed with HIV infection had not seen themselves as having been at risk (Lindsay *et al.*, 1991).

Africa

Summary Epidemiological studies in Africa, where HIV is transmitted primarily through heterosexual contact, found that HIV seroprevalence and incidence rates were higher in adolescent females than males. Risk factors for HIV included multiple sex partners, history of sexually transmitted disease and living in an urban area. Among females, the highest HIV prevalence and incidence was often reported in adolescents or women in their early twenties.

Seroprevalence / incidence surveys conducted in Africa

Tanzania In a 1990-91 seroprevalence survey in Mwanza region, HIV was more common in younger women than younger men. Among people aged 15-24 years, HIV seroprevalence in women exceeded that for men in 3 separate groups; urban (females 16.5%, males 5.4%); "roadside" or semi-urban (10.7% v 1.2%) and village (3.6% v 0.6%). Only above the age of 35 years was male seroprevalence greater than female's. Risk factors for HIV, primarily transmitted through heterosexual contact, included multiple sex partners, history of STD and, for the rural population, travel to the urban area (Barongo *et al.*, 1992).

A study in Kagera region north west Tanzania, found that in 1987-88 HIV *incidence* in females aged 15-19 years (8.3 per 1,000 person years) exceeded that for males (0.0 per 1,000). Furthermore, among the 783 females aged 15-54 years in the study, the highest age-specific HIV incidence was in younger women, aged 20-24 years (31.0 per 1,000). For the 533 males, age-specific incidence was highest among the slightly older 25-34 years old (30.9 per 1,000) (Killewo *et al.*, 1993).

Among blood donors in south-west Tanzania overall seroprevalence in 1988-91 was similar for males (6.3%) and females (6.2%). However, among adolescent donors aged 15-19 years, 7.3% of the females but only 1.6% of the males tested positive for HIV antibody. Women in their twenties also had a higher seroprevalence than men; only above the age of 30 years did male exceed female rates. Urban blood donors had the highest seroprevalence (16.6% at age 15-24 years), semi-urban an intermediate rate (6.8%) and rural donors the lowest (3.0%) (Soderberg, *et al.*, 1994).

In a 1989-90 population based survey in North Mara district, Tanzania, HIV seroprevalence in adolescent females aged 15-19 years was 5.1% compared with 1.2% in males of the same age. As in other studies, women in their twenties also had a higher seroprevalence than men. Urban adolescents (both male and female) had higher seroprevalence than their rural counterparts (Shao *et al.*, 1994)

More than 2,000 women aged 15-48 years attending three family planning clinics in Dar-es-Salaam in 1991-92 were tested for HIV; overall seroprevalence was 11.5% (262/2,289). Although HIV seroprevalence was lowest (4.2%) in adolescent females aged 15-19 years, women who reported first sexual intercourse *before* the age of 20 years had twice the seroprevalence of women whose first sexual intercourse was at a later age. Thus, in this study, adolescent age at first intercourse appeared to be an independent risk factor for HIV infection in women (Kapiga *et al.*, 1994).

Table 6
Africa, HIV seroprevalence surveys

	Year	Age group (years)	Sex	Seroprevalence per 1000 (number HIV positive /number tested)		Reference
›ulation	1990-1991	15-24	M (urban)	54	(12/222)	Barongo et al 1992
			F (urban)	165	(38/245)	
rs	1988-1991	15-19	M	16	(2/129)	Soderberg et a 1994
			F	73	(9/124)	
›ulation a)	1989-1990	15-19	M	12	(3/254)	Shao et al 1994
			F	51	(24/475)	
ning lers am)	1991-1992	15-19	F	42	(8/191)	Kapiga et al 1994
›ulation	1989-1990	13-19	M (urban)	0	(0/29)	Wawer et al 1991
			F (urban)	500	(20/40)	
›ulation	1986	16-25	M+F (urban)	170	(29/170)	Rwandan HIV seroprevalence study group 1
			M+F (rural)	12	(2/168)	

Uganda A 1989-90 survey in Rakai district, south west Uganda, revealed a higher overall seroprevalence among women than men. As in other African studies, this differential was largely due to higher female seroprevalence at younger ages (13-19 and 20-34 years). For example, HIV seroprevalence in urban adolescents aged 13-19 years living in trading centres was 50% (20/40) for females, but 0% (0/29) for males. While seroprevalence in rural areas was lower than in trading centres, the female rate still exceeded the male's (9 v 1%). HIV infection was predominantly transmitted by heterosexual contact and was associated with multiple partners (Wawer *et al.*, 1991).

HIV seroprevalence in Masaka district, south west Uganda was higher in females aged 15-24 years than males of the same age in November 1990 (13 v 5%). During the following 12 months, HIV seroincidence rates in males and females aged 13-24 years were not significantly different (12.8 and 10.6 per 1,000 person years) in marked contrast to the elevated rate seen in males aged 25-54 years (12.3 per 1,000 person years for males v 3.0 per 1,000 person years for females). Heterosexual contact was the principal mode of transmission. Over the 12 month follow up, HIV accounted for 75% of deaths among adolescents and adults in their early twenties (Mulder, 1994).

Rwanda In a nationwide survey conducted in Rwanda in 1986, seroprevalence in urban residents aged 16-25 was 17.0%. Seroprevalence was greater in females than males particularly in 16-25 years olds, although age – and sex – specific rates were not provided by the authors. HIV seroprevalence in rural residents was lower (16-25 years, 1.2%) and showed no sex difference (Rwandan HIV Seroprevalence Study Group, 1989).

Among antenatal clinic attenders in a semi-rural area near Butawe town, younger women (<30 years) had higher seroprevalence than older women. Seroprevalence in women under 20 years was 11.2%, similar to that seen in women in their twenties. More striking, perhaps, was that 20% of women who first became pregnant before their eighteenth birthday were seropositive compared with 10% who first became pregnant at or above this age. Age at first pregnancy remained a risk for HIV in multivariate analysis, as did history of STD and number of sexual partners (Chao 1994).

In a seroincidence survey in Kigali among 216 parturient women, 20 seroconverted during follow up between 1988-92 (3.5 per 100 woman years). This did not vary by maternal age. For females aged 15-19 years, the incidence was 4.3 per 100 woman years. None of the woman who seroconverted had received blood products or transfusions (Leroy, 1994).

Other countries

Summary Epidemiological studies in other countries have also confirmed that socially and economically disadvantaged teenagers – be they sex workers, the homeless or the poor – are at high risk for HIV infection. But they have also revealed that, among adolescents age and sex differentials HIV vary between communities and countries.

In *Argentina,* 30% (127/606) of adolescent "street youths" aged 13-20 years in security institutions in Buenos Aires were HIV positive in 1988-92. HIV prevalence was higher among males (24.6%; 119/483) than females (6.5%; 8/123) although this was confounded in part by injecting drug use which was more common in men than women. Among injecting drug users seroprevalence was in fact similar for males (56%; 82/146) and females (57%; 8/14). Among non injecting drug users, however, male seroprevalence (11%; 37/337) exceeded female's (0%; 0/109) (Libonatti *et al.* 1994).

In northern *Thailand,* 65% (177/273) of female commercial sex workers (CSW) were HIV positive in a 1992 seroprevalence survey. Nearly half the sex workers were teenagers or just twenty years old. Seroprevalence was equally high among adolescent CSWs (66.0%) as those aged 21 years and above (64.5%). History of STD, ethnicity and charging a low price for services were significantly associated with HIV infection (Celentano *et al.,* 1994). A further study in northern Thailand found that 60% of female CSWs were 20 years old or under and, because of the high turnover rate, new teenage girls were continually being recruited for commercial sex work (Sawanpanyalert *et al.,* 1994).

Among 2,417 male military conscripts aged 19-23 years in northern *Thailand,* 12.0% (289) were HIV positive when they were recruited in 1991. It was not known when the conscripts were infected, but many would have been teenagers at the time. HIV infection was strongly associated with heterosexual activity, number of lifetime sex partners, sex with female CSWs and history of STD. Sex between males and injecting drug use were uncommon and not associated with HIV infection (Nelson *et al.,* 1993).

In a 1992 population-based survey in 5 northern *Thailand* villages, HIV seroprevalence among 15-19 year old male adolescents (23.5%, 4/17) exceeded that in females of the same age (0%, 0/13). A male excess was also seen among 20-29 year olds; male seroprevalence 25.6% (11/43), female's 4.0% (3/70). This stands in marked contrast to the pattern seen among adolescents in African surveys where HIV seroprevalence among females exceeded the rate of males, or the USA where male and female rates were often similar. In the Thai study, between 1990-92 the highest 2 year seroincidence rate in males was recorded among 15-19 year old adolescents (11.8%). No females were infected at this age (Nelson *et al.,* 1994). This epidemiological pattern again contrasts markedly with that in other countries where adolescent males often had the lowest incidence and seroprevalence in men.

In a study among 210 male injecting drug users in northern *Malaysia,* 30% tested positive for HIV antibody. Although seroprevalence increased with age and was lowest among adolescents, nonetheless 9% of injecting drug users under the age of 20 years were seropositive. Nearly 20% of adolescents who had been injecting for 2-3 years were infected with HIV (Singh & Crofts, 1993.)

A seroprevalence study was conducted in Palermo, *Italy,* among more than 800 injecting drug users attending the AIDS Regional Reference Center between 1985 and 1990. Overall, 49% (332/678) of the males and 68% (89/134) of the females were HIV positive. In univariate analysis, seroprevalence increased with both duration of drug use and age, although even among adolescents aged 14-19 years 20% of the males (13/64) and 27% (3/11) of the females tested positive for HIV. After adjusting for number of years of drug use, however, age became a protective factor – adolescents and people in their early twenties had a greater chance of being infected with HIV than older drug users, probably because younger people were not using safer injecting techniques (Romano *et al.*, 1992).

In *Mexico* City, over 2000 gay and bisexual men were tested for HIV at the AIDS National Center, a free confidential testing and counselling service in 1988-89. Overall 31.0% (717/2314) were HIV positive. Although seroprevalence rose steadily with age to 36% in men aged 25 years and over, nonetheless 16% (31/191) of adolescents aged 13-19 years were HIV positive. HIV infection was associated with sexual practice, number of partners and (inversely) with educational attainment (Hernandez *et al.*, 1992).

CONCLUSION

Several clear messages concerning HIV infection in adolescence have emerged from the epidemiological studies and HIV/AIDS surveillance data presented in this chapter.

Firstly, in many communities, females are equally if not more likely to acquire HIV in adolescence than males. In Africa, where HIV is transmitted primarily through heterosexual contact, seroprevalence and incidence rates were higher in female than male adolescents. In the United States of America, male and female adolescents had similar HIV seroprevalence in marked contract to the elevated rates seen in men at older ages. Secondly, adolescent males with sexually-acquired HIV in the United States of America and Europe predominantly reported sex with other men as their risk for HIV. Thirdly, in Europe approximately half the injecting drug users with AIDS were infected during adolescence. For no other exposure category was the proportion infected in adolescence so high. Disadvantaged youth, blacks and Hispanics in the USA were at high risk of acquiring HIV infection. Indeed the close link between social deprivation and HIV infection reported among adults in the USA was also found in adolescents. Finally seroprevalence rates among teenage girls in Africa and teenage boys in Thailand generally exceeded rates among adults although the reverse pattern was seen in the USA and Europe.

What are the implications of these findings for HIV prevention and education? Sex between men accounted for most cases of sexually acquired HIV infection among teenage males in the UK. Many of these boys would have been infected in the 1980s and early 1990s at a time when sex between men was still illegal for teenagers in the UK. Although the age of consent was reduced to 18 years in 1993, the stigma that surrounds homosexual relations and the fact that such relations are still illegal under the age of 18 years must raise questions about the extent to which sex between men is discussed openly in schools and other places. Yet not to do so may continue to place gay teenagers at high risk for HIV through unsafe sexual practices. Since the age of consent varies between European countries and American states, opportunities for prevention among teenagers will differ across continents. Clearly interventions at an early age are required in the UK and elsewhere since the risk of acquiring HIV infection increases rapidly through adolescence.

Teenage girls must be alerted to the fact that they may face a greater risk than teenage boys of acquiring HIV infection through heterosexual contact and that overall women with AIDS are more likely to be infected during adolescence than men. Strategies for prevention will need to be tailored to individual localities, be it an African trading centre or a hostel for the homeless in New York. Further research is also urgently required to explain the differential risk of HIV infection experienced by male and female adolescents reporting heterosexual contact as their exposure.

For Europe as a whole, approximately half the injecting drug users with AIDS were infected with HIV during adolescence. For no other exposure category was the proportion infected during adolescence so high. Injecting drug use in an illegal activity in most if not all countries, with creates immense problems for education and prevention in this domain. Nonetheless, successful interventions among adult injecting drug users would suggest that effective programmes can also be established among teenagers. Not to do so will place European adolescents who inject drugs at an extremely high risk for HIV. The fact that disadvantaged adolescents and homeless youth are at particularly high risk for HIV infection requires urgent intervention. Although this phenomenon has been primarily documented in the USA, it seems likely that a similar pattern will also prevail in European countries.

A diagnosis of AIDS during adolescence, although less common in teenagers than asymptomatic HIV infection, reflects exposure to HIV at a very early age indeed. As the number of AIDS cases due to contaminated blood products diminishes among teenagers, sexual intercourse and injecting drug use during and even before adolescence will assume increasing importance as a risk for HIV infection during the delicate transition from childhood to adult life. Epidemiological surveillance needs to be strengthened and interventions to prevent HIV transmission among adolescents developed so that this transition can be as smooth as is humanly possible.

ACKNOWLEDGEMENTS

I would like to thank Dr Ahilya Noone, PHLS Communicable Disease Surveillance Centre, London for providing HIV and AIDS surveillance data for the UK and Europe, Melanie Weerasuria, PHLS Communicable Disease Surveillance Centre, London for her expert data processing, Elaine Harris for meticulously typing the tables, Robert Bor for his valuable support and Lorraine Sherr for her infinite patience.

REFERENCES

Allen, D.M., Lehman, S.J., Green, T.A. *et al.* (1994) HIV infection among homeless adults and runaway youth, United States, 1989-1992, *AIDS*, **8**: 1593-1598.

Barongo, L.R., Borgdorff, M.W., Mosha, F.F. *et al.* (1992) The epidemiology of HIV-1 infection in urban areas, roadside settlements and rural villages in Mwanza Region, Tanzania, *AIDS*, **6**: 1521-1528.

Berrios, D.C., Hearst, N., Coates, T.J. *et al.* (1993) HIV antibody testing among those at risk for infection, the national AIDS behavioural surveys, *Journal of the American Medical Association*, **270**: 1576-1580.

Bowler, S., Sheon, A.R, D'Angelo, L.J., Vermund, S.H. (1992) HIV and AIDS among adolescents in the United States: increasing risk in the 1990s, *Journal of Adolescence*, **15**: 345-371.

Burke, D.S., Brundage, J.F., Goldenbaum, M. *et al.* (1990) Human immunodeficiency virus infections in teenagers, seroprevalence among applicants for the US military service, *Journal of the American Medical Association*, **263**: 2074-2077.

CDC (1992) Publicly funded HIV counseling and testing - United States 1991, *Morbidity and Mortality Weekly Report*, **41**: 613-617.

CDC (1994) HIV/AIDS surveillance report, US HIV and AIDS cases reported through June 1994, US Department of Health and Human Services, *Atlanta*, **6**: (No. 1), 9, 10, 12, 13.

Celentano, D.D., Akarasewi, P., Sussman, L. *et al.* (1994) HIV-infection among lower class commercial sex workers in Chiang Mai, Thailand, *AIDS*, **8**: 533-537.

Chao, A., Bulterys, M., Musanganire, F. *et al.* (1994) Risk factors associated with prevalent HIV-1 infection along pregnant women in Rwanda, *International Journal of Epidemiology*, **23**: 371-380.

Conway, G.A., Epstein, M.R., Hayman, C.R. *et al.* (1993) Trends in HIV prevalence among disadvantaged youth, survey results from a national job training program 1988 through 1992, *Journal of the American Medical Association*, **269**: 2887-2889.

Cowan, D.N., Pomerantz, R.S., Wann, Z.F. *et al.* (1990) Human immunodeficiency virus infection among members of the Reserve Components of the US army; prevalence, incidence, and demographic characteristics, *Journal of Infectious Diseases*, **162**: 827-836.

Cowan, D.N., Brundage, J.F., Pomerantz, R.S., (1994) The incidence of HIV infection among men in the United States Army Reserve Components, 1985-1991, *AIDS*, **8**: 505-511.

D'Angelo, L.J., Getson, P.R., Luban, N.L.C., Gayle, H.D. (1991) Human immunodeficiency virus infection in urban adolescents: can we predict who is at risk? *Pediatrics*, **88**: 982-986.

D'Angelo, L.J. (1994) Adolescents and HIV infection: a clinician's perspective, *Acta Paediatrica Supplement*, **400**: 88-94.

European Centre for the Epidemiological Monitoring of AIDS (1994) *AIDS surveillance in Europe, Quarterly Report no.* **43**: 30 September 1994.

Friedman, L.S., Goodman, E., (1992) Adolescents at risk for HIV infection, *Primary Care*, **19**: 171-190.

Futterman, D., Hein, K., Reuben, N. *et al.* (1993) Human immunodeficiency virus-infected adolescents; the first 50 patients in a New York City program, *Pediatrics*, **91**: 730-735.

Gayle, H.D., Keeling, R.P., Garcia-Tunon, M., *et al.* (1990) Prevalence of the human immunodeficiency virus among university students, *New England Journal of Medicine*, **323**: 1538-1541.

Gayle, H.D., D'Angelo, L.J., (1991) Epidemiology of AIDS and HIV infection in adolescents, in Pediatric AIDS; the challenge of HIV infection in infants, children and adolescents, Pizzo PA and Wilfert CM (eds), Williams and Wilkins, Baltimore.

Hernandez, M., Uribe, P., Gortmaket, S. *et al.* (1992) Sexual behaviour and status for human immunodeficiency virus type 1 among homosexual and bisexual males in Mexico City, *American Journal of Epidemiology*, **135**: 883-894.

Kapiga, S.H., Shao, J.F., Lwihula, G.K., Hunter, D.J. (1994) Risk factors for HIV infection among women in Dar-es-Salaam, Tanzania, *Journal of Acquired Immune Deficiency Syndromes*, 7: 301-309.

Killewo, J.Z.J., Sandstrom, A., Bredberg Raden, U. *et al.* (1993) Incidence of HIV-1 infection among adults in the Kagera region of Tanzania, *International Journal of Epidemiology*, **22**: 528-536.

Killewo, J., Nyamuryekunge, K., Sandstrom, A. *et al.* (1990) Prevalence of HIV-1 infection in the Kagera region of Tanzania: a population-based study, *AIDS*, **4**: 1081-1085.

Leroy, V., van de Perre, P., Lepage, P. *et al.* (1994) Seroincidence of HIV-1 infection in African woman of reproductive age: a prospective cohort study in Kigali, Rwanda, 1988-1992, *AIDS*, **8**: 983-986.

Libonatti, O., Casaneuva, E., Avila, M.M. *et al.* (1994) HIV-1 and HBV infection in street youth lodged in security institutes of Buenos Aires, *Journal of Acquired Immune Deficiency Syndromes*, 7: 98-101.

Lindsay, M.K., Peterson, H.B., Willis., S. *et al.* (1991) Incidence and prevalence of human immunodeficiency virus infection in a prenatal population undergoing routine voluntary human immunodeficiency virus screening, July 1987 to June 1990, *American Journal of Obstetrics and Gynecology*, **165**: 961-964.

McNeil, J.G., Brundage, J.F., Gardner, L.I. *et al.* (1991) Trends of HIV seroconversion among young adults in the US army, 1985 to 1989, *Journal of the American Medical Association*, **265**: 1709-1714.

Melnick, S.L., Sherer, R., Louis, T.A., *et al.* (1994) Survival and disease progression according to gender of patients with HIV infection. The Terry Beirn Community Programs for Clinical Research on AIDS, *Journal of the American Medical Association*, **272**: 1915-1921.

Mulder, D.W., Nunn, A.J., Wagner, H.U. *et al.* (1994) HIV-1 incidence and HIV-1 associated mortality in a rural Ugandan population cohort, *AIDS*, **8**: 87-92.

Munoz, A., Wang, M.C., Bass, S. *et al.* (1989) Acquired immunodeficiency syndrome (AIDS)-free time after human immunodeficiency virus type 1 (HIV-1) seroconversion in homosexual men, Multicenter AIDS Cohort Study Group, *American Journal of Epidemiology*, **130**: 530-539.

Nelson, K.E., Celentano, D.D., Suprasert, S., *et al.* (1993) Risk factors of HIV infection among young adult men in northern Thailand, *Journal of the American Medical Association*, **270**: 955-960.

Noone, A., Durante, A.J., Brady A.R. *et al.* (1993) HIV infection in injecting drug users attending centres in England and Wales, 1990-1991, *AIDS*, 7: 1501-1507.

Novick, L.F., Berns, D., Stricof, R. *et al.* (1989) HIV seroprevalence in newborns in New York State, *Journal of the American Medical Association*, **261**: 1745-1750.

PHLS Communicable Disease Surveillance Centre (1995) AIDS and HIV-1 infection in the United Kingdom: monthly report, *Communicable Disease Report*, **5**: No. 3, 13-16.

Quinn, T.C., Glasser, D., Cannon, R.O. *et al.* (1988) Human Immunodeficiency virus infection among patients attending clinics for sexually transmitted diseases. *New England Journal of Medicine*, **318**: 197-203.

Quinn, T.C., Groseclose, S.L., Spence, M., *et al.* (1992) Evolution of the human immunodeficiency virus epidemic among patients attending sexually transmitted disease clinics: a decade of experience, *Journal of Infectious Diseases*, **165**: 541-544.

Romano, N., Vitale, F., Alesi, D.R., *et al.* (1992) The changing pattern of human immunodeficiency virus type 1 infection in intravenous drug users, Results of a six-year seroprevalence study in Palermo, Italy, *American Journal of Epidemiology*, **135**: 1189-1196.

Rwandan HIV Seroprevalence Study Group (1989) Nationwide community-based serological survey of HIV-1 and other human retrovirus infections in a Central African country, *Lancet*, **i**: 941-943.

St Louis, M.E., Rauch, K.J., Petersen, L.R., *et al.* (1990) Seroprevalence rates of human immunodeficiency virus infection at sentinel hospitals in the United States, *New England Journal of Medicine*, **323**: 213-218.

St Louis, M.E., Conway, G.A., Hayman, G.R., *et al.* (1991) Human immunodeficiency virus infection in disadvantaged adolescents, findings from the US Job Corps, *Journal of the American Medical Association*, **266**: 2387-2391.

Sawanpanyalert, P., Ungchusak, K, Thanprasertsuk, S., Akarasewi, P. (1994) HIV-1 seroconversion rates among female commercial sex workers, Chiang Mai, Thailand: a multi cross-sectional study, *AIDS*, **8**: 825-829.

Shao, J., Brubaker, G., Levin, A. *et al.* (1994) Population-based study of HIV-1 infection in 4086 subjects in northwest Tanzania, *Journal of Acquired Immune Deficiency Syndromes*, 7: 397-402.

Singh, S., Crofts, N. (1993) HIV infection among injecting drug users in north-east Malaysia, *AIDS Care*, **5**: 275-283.

Soderberg, S., Temihango, W., Kadate, C., *et al.* (1994) Prevalence of HIV-1 infection in rural, semi-urban and urban villages in southwest Tanzania: estimates from a blood-donor study, *AIDS*, **8**: 971-976.

Stricof, R.L., Kennedy, J.T., Nattell, T.C., Weisfuse, I.B., Novick, L.F. (1991) HIV seroprevalence in a facility for runaway and homeless adolescents, *American Journal of Public Health*, **81 (supplement)**: 50-53.

Wawer, M.J., Serwadda D., Musgrave, S.D. *et al.* (1991) Dynamics of spread of HIV-1 infection in a rural district of Uganda, *British Medical Journal*, **303**: 1303-1306.

Wendell, D.A., Onorato, I.M., McCray, E. *et al.* (1992) Youth at risk. Sex, drugs and human immunodeficiency virus, *American Journal of Diseases in Children*, **146**: 76-81.

4

AIDS Diagnoses in US Adolescents 1981-1993 : The Future Arrives

CHERYL A. KENNEDY & HAFTAN M. ECKHOLDT

INTRODUCTION

Data from the United States (US) AIDS Public Information Data Set (AIDSPIDS, 1995) provided by the Centers for Disease Control and Prevention (CDC), Atlanta, Georgia, are presented with the focus on the diagnoses (cases) of AIDS among US adolescents and young adults through 1993. The diagnoses of AIDS increase the most when individuals move from adolescence (13 to 19 years old) to young adulthood (20 to 24 years old). African Americans and Latino Americans are over represented among all Americans diagnosed with AIDS. More than one half of all diagnoses among the younger age groups are African Americans and Latino Americans. The proportion of AIDS diagnoses is growing among females and the heterosexual transmission group, so that women and men have similar or equal rates of diagnoses among African American and Latino American cases. The proportion of heterosexual transmissions is highest among younger African American diagnoses. These data suggest that adolescent African American and Latino American diagnoses were at a demographic epicenter of HIV at its most dynamic moment in 1993 justifying continued focused studies of those so affected. Trends and policy implications of these data are discussed. The rising tide of young adults infected and at risk demands that Public Health research and policy act innovatively, swiftly and decisively to implement disease prevention and health promotion.

EPIDEMIOLOGY

The following discussion includes analyses of trends in the US epidemiology of Acquired Immunodeficiency Syndrome (AIDS) in adolescents and young adults from 1981 through 1993 as taken from the AIDS Public Information Data Set (AIDSPIDS, 1995), a raw data set of AIDS diagnoses in the United States. These data are from the United States Department of Health and Human Services, at the Centers for Disease Control and Prevention (CDC) in Atlanta, Georgia, Further discussion will encompass the trends and policy implications of this analysis.

AGE

The age at diagnosis with AIDS in the US has had a stable distribution throughout the history of HIV in the United States. There is a ten fold increase in AIDS diagnoses from the adolescent age group (13-19), which makes up about 0.4% of all AIDS diagnoses, to the young adult age group (20-24), which makes up about 3.8% of all diagnoses. This trend can be found within each race group as well. Because most, if not all, of the 20 to 24 year old diagnoses (N=16,575), and a portion of the 25 to 29 year old diagnoses (N=65,071) (as December 1994, CDC, 1994a), are the result of adolescent exposures [factoring in an 8 year incubation period as described by Lui *et al.*, (1988) and Goedert *et al.*, (1989)], HIV goes through its greatest acceleration in transmission during adolescence (Des Jarlais *et al.*, 1990).

A RACIAL DISTRIBUTION

African American and Latino American cases have always been over represented among AIDS diagnoses in the US, and since 1984 the proportion of African American and Latino American cases of AIDS has been increasing steadily. African Americans make up about 12% of the US population, while African American diagnoses account for 33% of all AIDS cases. Furthermore, Latino Americans make up about 9% of the US population, yet they account for more than 17% of all AIDS diagnoses to date (Statistical Abstract of the US, 1992, CDC, 1994a). Asians and Pacific Islanders make up 2.9% of the US population and 0.68% of cumulative AIDS diagnoses; Native American Indians are approximately 0.8% of the population and 0.24% of AIDS diagnoses to date. The overall population of AIDS diagnoses accounted for by each race are reflected within each age group as well – African Americans and Latino Americans, combined, account for more than one half of all diagnoses in all age groups up through adulthood. Latinos and Asians and Pacific Islanders are the only race groups to report a steadily increasing proportion of total diagnoses each year since 1981. At no time did total diagnoses in the United States experience the 3 fold increase of Asians and Pacific Islander diagnoses from 1984 to 1985, or the 3 fold increase of Native American Indian diagnoses from 1985-1986. Further discussions of AIDS diagnoses by race are best made through the exploration of longitudinal changes within various subgroups within each race.

Table 1
Frequency of AIDS Diagnoses (%) by Race, Age Grop, and Year (AIDSPIDS, 1995).

Age	Race White		Black		Latino		A/PI		Nat AM		Total	
to 12	1	11%	6	67%	2	22%	0	0.00%	0	0.00%	9	2.
to 19	2	40%	2	40%	1	20%	0	0.00%	0	0.00%	5	1.
to 24	8	38%	10	48%	3	14%	0	0.00%	0	0.00%	21	5.
to 29	28	42%	27	40%	12	18%	0	0.00%	0	0.00%	67	16.
to 34	47	53%	26	29%	15	17%	0	0.00%	1	1.12%	89	22.
l ages	228	57%	110	28%	57	14%	1	0.25%	1	0.25%	398	
to 12	35	26%	67	49%	33	24%	2	1.46%	0	0.00%	137	1.
to 19	14	25%	26	47%	15	27%	0	0.00%	0	0.00%	55	0.
to 24	317	54%	172	29%	91	16%	4	0.68%	1	0.17%	586	5.
to 29	1075	55%	570	29%	293	15%	13	0.66%	1	0.05%	1956	16.
to 34	1637	56%	811	28%	448	15%	15	0.51%	4	0.14%	2918	24.
l ages	6957	59%	2961	25%	1712	15%	75	0.64%	10	0.09%	11728	
to 12	103	23%	219	48%	129	28%	2	0.44%	1	0.22%	455	1.
to 19	81	47%	61	35%	29	17%	1	0.58%	1	0.58%	173	0.
to 24	734	42%	594	34%	382	22%	8	0.46%	10	0.58%	1730	4.
to 29	3395	51%	1938	29%	1270	19%	45	0.67%	23	0.34%	6682	15.
to 34	5172	51%	3126	31%	1748	17%	60	0.59%	21	021%	10139	24.
l ages	22003	52%	12677	30%	7096	17%	295	0.70%	83	0.20%	42232	
to 12	84	17%	300	59%	116	23%	4	0.79%	0	0.00%	506	0.
to 19	99	29%	166	49%	71	21%	2	0.59%	1	0.29%	339	0.
to 24	739	32%	1046	45%	511	22%	20	0.86%	7	0.30%	2326	3.
to 29	3720	39%	3567	38%	2060	22%	66	0.70%	46	0.49%	9470	13.
to 34	6972	44%	5644	35%	3174	20%	129	0.81%	43	0.27%	15986	22.

Early in the epidemic, Whites accounted for about one half of all US adolescent diagnoses (13-19 years) and about one quarter of young adult diagnoses (20-24 years). **See Table 1.** In 1986, Whites accounted for about 46% of adolescent diagnoses and more than one half of all young adult diagnoses (20 to 24 as well as 25 to 29). By 1991, African Americans and Latino Americans combined, account for more than one half of all diagnoses in all age groups up through adulthood (30-34), and well over one half of the adolescent (58%) and young adult case (56%). Although it is well known that African American and Latino American cases are over represented, these data show that African American and Latino American adolescents are a growing majority of diagnoses within their age group.

GENDER RATIO

Across all age groups, the ratio of female-to-male diagnoses is consistently lower among African American and Latino American and Native American diagnoses,

Table 2
Female:Male Diagnoses by Race, Age Group, and Year (AIDSPIDS, 1995)

Year	Age	White	Black	Latino	A/PI	Nat Am	Total
1981	1 to 12	0	01:01	01:01			1:1.5
	13 to 19		0				1:0.8
	20 to 24	01:07	01:04	01:02			01:04
	25 to 29	01:27	01:08	01:03			1:4.25
	30 to 34		1:3.3	01:14		0	1:8.6
	all ages	01:27	1:4.7	01:05	0	0	1:9.1
1985	1 to 12	1:0.8	1:0.76	1:1.2			1:1.2
	13 to 19	1:3.7	1:4.2				1:0.9
	20 to 24	1:21.6	1:4.7	1:3.3			1:5.9
	25 to 29	1:24.6	1:3.9	1:6.5			1:8
	30 to 34	1:30.5	1:4.8	1:7.96	01:14	01:01	1:8.9
	all ages	1:27.1	1:5.04	1:7.8	01:18	01:04	1:11.4
1989	1 to 12	1:1.6	1:1.1	1:1	01:01	0	1:0.8
	13 to 19	1:3.8	1:1.3	1:2.6			1:1.2
	20 to 24	1:7.8	1:2.9	1:3.6	1:1.6	01:04	1:2.4
	25 to 29	1:14.4	1:3.4	1:4.6	01:01	1:4.7	1:4.3
	30 to 34	1:17.4	1:3.7	1:5.7	01:19	01:20	1:6.5
	all ages	1:16.4	1:3.8	1:5.5	1:10.3	01:06	1:7.4
1993	1 to 12	01:01	01:01	1:0.8	01:03		1:0.8
	13 to 19	1:6.6	1:0.6	1:1.4	1:		1:1
	20 to 24	1:3.9	1:1.6	1:2.4	1:5.6	01:06	1:1.3
	25 to 29	1:6.8	1:2.4	1:3.9	01:10	1:5.6	1:2.3
	30 to 34	1:9.3	1:2.7	1:3.9	1:10.7	1:4.4	1:3.9
	all ages	1:9.6	1:2.9	1:4.1	1:8.4	1:4.7	1:4.7
TOTAL		1:13.6	1:3.4	1:5.1	1:8.9	1:5.4	1:6.2

note: "all ages" includes infant through geriatric, total includes unknown compared to Whites and Asian and Pacific Islanders. This suggests that men and women are at more similar risk for HIV exposure among African Americans, Latinos and Native Americans. The female-to-male ratio is also lower among younger age groups in each race group, and lowest among African Americans. **Table 2** shows that HIV has been increasing rapidly among women over the past decade. Furthermore, younger women are at greater risk for HIV than are older women, and younger African American women are at risk equal to that of African American men.

TRANSMISSION GROUPS: AGE, RACE & TIME

Table 3 focuses on HIV transmission groups and their interactions with age and race over time. In order to focus prediction within a single group which has similar risk behaviors, the discussion will be limited to two sexual transmission groups: men who have sex with men (MSM) and heterosexuals. Studies of adolescent injecting drug use (IDU) suggest that rates may be as low as 2%-5% in large sample surveys (CDC, 1990), 0.5% in smaller samples focusing on large cities (Des Jarlais *et al.*, 1990), and some researchers see IDU rates as low as 0.1% (Henggeler, *et al.*, 1992).

The distribution of sexual transmission groups within each age group (**Table 3**) shows that heterosexual transmission is most pronounced among younger age groups. In 1981, there were no AIDS diagnoses attributable to heterosexual transmission below the age of 25 years. By 1993, more adolescent diagnoses (age 13 to 19) were attributed to heterosexual (26%) than MSM (15%) transmissions. For all older age groups, MSM transmissions have been dropping over time: in 1985, MSM transmissions accounted for 61% of 20-24, 25-29, and 30-34 year old diagnoses; by 1993, MSM transmissions accounted for 42% of 20-24 year old diagnoses, and 50% of 25-29 year old diagnoses, 49% of 30-34 year old diagnoses.

Analyses of data on race and sex within the heterosexual transmission group shows that African American adolescents have had more heterosexual diagnoses than MSM diagnoses since 1989 (Latino Heterosexuals/MSM since 1992), with almost 2 heterosexual diagnoses for each MSM diagnosis by 1993 (57 Heterosexual versus 30 MSM). The ratio of female to male diagnoses by race within heterosexual transmissions suggests that women represent the majority (67%) of heterosexual transmissions. In every race group, women make up at least 65% of the heterosexual diagnoses regardless of age and in the case of White, African American and Latino American adolescents, females are nearly 100% of the diagnoses (AIDSPIDS, 1995).

A second trend can be seen in heterosexual transmissions – African American diagnoses make up the majority (52%) of all heterosexual cases to date – while Latino Americans and Whites share most of the remaining heterosexual transmissions (AIDSPIDS, 1995). The uniqueness of African American heterosexual diagnoses is especially apparent among African American adolescent (age 13-19) males, who show the highest cumulative frequency (18 cases), compared to Latino American male adolescents (8 cases), White male adolescents (5 cases), and Asian and Pacific Islander male adolescents (0) or Native American male adolescents (1 case) (data not shown, AIDSPIDS, 1995). The exceptionally high rate of African

American heterosexual male diagnoses is reflected in every other comparison in which African American heterosexual diagnoses (male and female) outnumber the White and Latino American heterosexual diagnoses by at least 2 to 1.

Table 3
AIDS Diagnoses for transmission group by age group and year (AIDSPIDS, 1995)

		Transmission						All Trans-
Age	Year	MSM		Het		Other		missions
1 to 12	1981	0	0%	0	0%	9	100%	9
	1985	0	0%	0	0%	137	100%	137
	1989	0	0%	0	0%	455	100%	455
	1993	0	0%	0	0%	506	100%	506
	all years	0	0%	0	0%	3786	100%	3786
13 to 19	1981	3	60%	0	0%	2	40%	5
	1985	20	36%	2	4%	33	60%	55
	1989	40	23%	29	17%	104	60%	173
	1993	52	15%	87	26%	200	59%	339
	all years	417	21%	374	19%	1174	60%	1965
20 to 24	1981	10	48%	1	5%	10	48%	21
	1985	355	61%	33	6%	198	34%	586
	1989	906	52%	184	11%	640	37%	1730
	1993	979	42%	477	21%	870	37%	2326
	all years	8110	49%	2302	14%	6163	37%	16575
25 to 29	1981	33	49%	1	1%	33	49%	67
	1985	1192	61%	60	3%	704	36%	1956
	1989	3932	59%	435	7%	2315	35%	6682
	1993	4745	50%	1349	14%	3376	36%	9470
	all years	36358	56%	5864	9%	22894	35%	65071
30 to 34	1981	54	61%	0	0%	35	39%	89
	1985	1776	61%	66	2%	1076	37%	2918
	1989	5685	56%	479	5%	3975	39%	10139
	1993	7863	49%	1657	10%	6466	40%	15986
	all years	55244	54%	7025	7%	40553	39%	102822
TOTAL	all years/ ages	228954	52%	31663	7%	180911	41%	441528

Rates of heterosexual HIV transmissions continued to rise through 1993 and were higher for African Americans (20 per 100,000) and Latino Americans (10 per 100,000) than for Whites (1 per 100,000), Asian/Pacific Islanders (1 per 100,000) and American Indians/Alaskan Natives (2 per 100,000). (CDC, 1994b). Since 1992, HIV infection is the number one cause of death in African Americans aged 25-44 years (for 1992: n=8,456; rate=83 per 100,000 population) and the fifth leading cause of death in ages 15-24 years (for 1992: n=286; rate=5.4 per 100,000 population) (CDC, 1995a). In fourteen years, over a half million cases of AIDS in the US have been diagnosed by the end of 1995 and 62% have died. (CDC, 1995b).

SOCIAL BACKDROP

The implications of the epidemiology of AIDS diagnoses and HIV-related sex behaviours in American adolescents must be interpreted in a broad societal and demographic context which includes an understanding of diverse ethno-cultural and other social reference group influences. The age of onset of sexual activity in the US is decreasing, the number of lifetime sex partners at each age is increasing, and the use of condoms is dangerously low. (Bachrach & Horn, 1988; Orr 1991; CDC, 1992; Stiffman *et al.*, 1994; Stanton *et al.*, 1994). These HIV-related behaviours portend continued high-risk for US adolescents, particularly against the backdrop of a culture which is clearly ambivalent about teen sex despite the evidentiary representation of actual sexual activity and exchange of body fluids embodied in the fact that over 1 million American teenage females have become pregnant each year from 1980-1990 (CDC, 1993). Writers since the late nineteen-eighties have realized that the trend in HIV incidence and AIDS diagnoses in adolescents pointed toward an adolescent wave of the HIV epidemic. (Hein, 1989; Vermund, 1989).

When considering the trends and direction of the epidemic, statisticians and epidemiologists have warned that although statistical ideas and approaches have contributed greatly to an understanding of transmission factors, strategies for prevention, description of the natural history of HIV infection, and clinical trial designs, there are many pitfalls and a naive approach can seriously mislead policy makers (Brookmeyer & Gail, 1994). In the case of the adolescent wave of the epidemic, it seems that the future has arrived.

Although pregnancy and acquisition of sexually transmitted diseases (STD), including HIV, may be the result of some of the same behaviour, the outcome differs greatly and different strategies are required to mediate outcome. For example, obviously, mere use of oral contraceptive agents does not protect from disease. And, though the pregnancy outcome may seem remote at the time of coitus, surely, the impact of a disease state 10 years in the future must seem even more distant to a healthy adolescent. More recent studies of sexual practices and intentions of pre-adolescent and early adolescent low-income urban African-Americans and Latinos since 1991 continued to confirm early coitus, multiple partners and low condom use rates (Eckholdt, 1994; Stanton *et al.*, 1994; Ford *et al.*, 1995).

It is now known, that to change some factors which influence first intercourse for adolescent males, profound changes in the way society is structured may be required. As social welfare programmes shrink (since government is less inclined to provide financial benefits for the poor), more single mothers will be required to work and thus, particularly among African Americans, place their sons at risk for early initiation into sexual activity (Ku *et al.*, 1993).

It is known that youngsters need confidence and a feeling of efficacy in order to use condoms (Mahoney *et al.*, 1995), and despite recent findings that substance use may be declining among some of America's youth, there is concern that the emphasis placed on resisting drug use may have diverted needed attention away from resisting early, unwanted or unprotected sex (Levy *et al.*, 1993). The necessary broad-based health promotion activities are required among the groups least likely to receive them.

As the HIV epidemic continues to ascend globally, the sexually active young continue to be the most vulnerable. Without effective antimicrobial intervention, efforts aimed at the behavioural components of acquisition and transmission must remain as the primary interventions for health professionals. Most US infections of HIV in adolescents to date have been in urban youth, but it may be that the epidemic has spread silently (and largely, untested) to other geographic, ex-urban areas where awareness and risk perception may be less acute.

Unfortunately, even knowledge and concern about risky activity does not translate into behavioural change for US adolescents. (Maticka-Tyndale, 1991; Skurnick *et al.,* 1991; CDC, 1992). Recent studies of college students reveal multiple risk behaviours despite high levels of perceived susceptibility to HIV and other STDs (Mahoney *et al.,* 1995). Approaches must be developmentally, culturally and socially relevant. Further, gender roles and issues of economic empowerment must be addressed if condom use or abstinence are to become widespread among youth as disease prevention measures (du Guerny & Sjoberg, 1993; Stanton, 1994). Out-of-school and disadvantaged youth, particularly females, are highest risk for acquiring HIV (Conway *et al.,* 1993; St. Louis, 1991). Competing interest may make it difficult for poor adolescents, especially females to give HIV the attention it demands for behavioural change to be effected. Urban and suburban youth who report psychological problems, adverse life circumstances (familial disruption, parental discord, economic hardship, crime) have higher involvement in high-risk behaviours, including substance use (Walter *et al.,* 1991).

POLICY IMPLICATIONS

Strategies that impact those teens who are outside the mainstream are crucial. All teens experience tremendous shifts in biological and cognitive functioning, while simultaneously experimenting with a wide array of sexual, moral and economic choices. Examining ways to empower the disenfranchised youth (many of whom are the off-spring of marginalized urban adults whose ranks are being decimated by AIDS) will be paramount in attempting to stem the advances of this epidemic.

Data and information on effective programmes continue to expand. Recommendations have been made to increase condom availability to youth and strategies known to increase condom use have been elucidated for some groups (Jemmott *et al.,* 1992; Jemmott & Jemmott, 1992; Ku *et al.,* 1993; Levy *et al.,* 1993; Mahoney *et al.,* 1995; Warden *et al.,* 1995; Committee on Adolescence, 1995). However, progressive and practical working knowledge is not applied across the board and many groups remain unstudied. Surely, information communication and availability of disease prevention methods need to be more widely utilized. An early education policy which takes necessary risks to teach and encourage youth to find the ways to make difficult cultural shifts must be promoted and undertaken. Innovative, problem-solving research must continue. It is generally agreed that integrated approaches which can impact multiple risk behaviours and their complicated inter-relationships are most successful and must be introduced early in school curricula. Reinforcement and continuing education are essential for success (Jemmott *et al.*, 1992). Further, specific approaches and interventions must be designed for marginal sub-groups which may vary greatly from locale to locale. Widespread, continuous and on-going education and prevention programs will require the continuous and on-going commitment of resources and motivation from communities and government.

A contemporary strategy by du Guerny and Sjoberg is based on their analysis of gender relations and the world-wide HIV epidemic (1993). They conclude that the health perspective must be broadened to include a wide ecological approach, including gender analysis of the socio-economic and cultural causes and effects of the epidemic. Globally, the spread of HIV is primarily heterosexual and women have the highest risk. Persons of color are disproportionately affected.

Any cohort with specific vulnerability based on economics and social circumstances must be exactingly addressed within their own cultural boundaries, such that behavioural change messages might be effective. Runaway youth, substances users, teens with psychological distress, teens who do not exhibit stereotypic sex roles, the impoverished and those with no social support are most at-risk and most difficult to reach. Even when successful strategies have been identified, avenues for dissemination and broad application are difficult (Rotheram-Bonus, 1995).

Throughout the world an entire future generation is at risk for HIV and its attendant morbidity and mortality. Youngsters of colour, particularly females and those at economic disadvantage are most susceptible. In areas of the world where there is political or social unrest or instability, the risk expands. As refugee populations continue to grow world-wide and social order is disrupted, it is less likely that practical public health measures, which could have a positive impact on adolescent behaviours, will be implemented.

While the US health care access and delivery system lurches toward an awkward new embrace of the marketplace, the young and poor remain in danger of further disenfranchisement. In addition to traditional settings and approaches, policies and programmes need to deploy creative and far-reaching strategies for health promotion. Yet, the larger question remains: In the absence of vast systemic socio-political and economic change regarding the status of girls, women minorities and the fostering of adolescent autonomy, will any message be effective?

REFERENCES

AIDS Public Information Data Set (AIDSPIDS) through December 1993 (1995) [computer software] Atlanta, GA: U.S. Centers for Diseases Control and Prevention, Division of HIV/AIDS. Inquiries (404) 639-2020.

Bachrach, C.A., & Horn, M.C. (1988) Sexual activity among U.S. women of reproductive age. *Amer J Pub Health*, 78: 320-321.

Brookmeyer, R., & Gail, M.H. (1994) *AIDS Epidemiology: A Quantitative Approach*. New York: Oxford University Press.

Centers for Disease Control and Prevention. (1990) HIV related knowledge and behaviors among high school students – selected U.S. sites, 1989. *Morbidity and Mortality Weekly report*, **39**: 385-397.

Centers for Disease Control and Prevention. (1992) Sexual behavior among high school students – United States, 1990. *Morbidity and Mortality Weekly Report*, **40**: 1-3.

Centers for Disease Control and Prevention. (1993) Surveillance for pregnancy and birth rates among teenagers by state – United States 1980 & 1990. *Morbidity and Mortality Weekly Report*, **42**:1.

Centers for Disease Control and Prevention. (1994a) *HIV/AIDS Surveillance Report*, **6**: 1-39.

Centers for Disease Control and Prevention. (1994b) Heterosexually Acquired AIDS-United States, 1993. *Morbidity and Mortality Weekly Report*, **43**: 155-160.

Centers for Disease Control and Prevention. (1995a) Advance Report of Final Mortality Statistics, 1992. *Monthly Vital Statistics Report*, **43**, (66 Suppl): 30.

Centers for Disease Control and Prevention. (1995b) AIDS Cases in US Since '81: 501,310. *CDC National AIDS Clearinghouse* (Originator: aidsnews@cdcnac.aspensys.com 11/27/95), Information, Inc., Bethesda, Maryland, USA.

Committee on Adolescence, Council on Child and Adolescent Health, American Academy of Pediatrics. (1995) Condom Availability for Youth. *Pediatrics*, **95**: 281-285.

Conway, G.A., Epstein, M.R., Hayman, C.R., *et al.* (1993) Trends in HIV Prevalence Among Disadvantaged Youth; Survey Results from a National Job Training Program, 1988 Through 1992. *Journal American Medical Association*, **269**: 2887-2889.

Des Jarlais, D.C., Ehrhardt, A.A., Fullilove, M.T., Hein, *et al.* (1990) AIDS and adolescents. In H.G. Miller, C.F. Turner, & Moses, L.E. Moses (Eds.), *AIDS: The second decade* (chap 3). Washington, D.C.: National Academy Press.

du Guerny, J. and Sjoberg, E. (1993) Inter-relationship between gender relations and the HIV/AIDS epidemic: some possible considerations for policies and programmes. *AIDS*,7:1027-1034.

Eckholdt, H.M. (1994) Ecological Prediction of HIV Risk Behaviors Among African American and Latino Adolescents in an AIDS Epicenter. Dissertation Abstracts International, 55-04B, (UnM) AAI 9422844.

Ford, K., Rubinstein, S., and Norris, A. (1994) Sexual Behavior and Condom Use Among Urban, Low-Income, African-American and Hispanic Youth. *AIDS Education and Prevention*, **6**: 219-229.

Goedert, J.J., Kessler, C.M., Aledot, L.M. *et al.* (1989) A prospective study of human immunodeficiency virus type 1 infection and the development of AIDS in subjects with hemophilia. *New England Journal Medicine*, **321**: 1141-1148.

Henggeler, S.W., Melton, G.B., & Rodrigue, J.R. (1992) *Pediatric and adolescent AIDS*. New York: Sage.

Hein, K. (1989) Commentary on Adolescent Acquired Immunodeficiency Syndrome: The Next Wave of the Human Immunodeficiency Virus Epidemic? *J of Pediatrics*, 114: 144-149.

Jemmott, L.S. & Jemmott J.B. (1992) Increasing Condom-Use Intentions Among Sexually Active Black Adolescent Women. *Nursing Research*, **41**: 273-279.

Jemmott, J.B., Jemmott, L.S., & Fong, G.T. (1992) Reductions in HIV risk-associated behaviors among black male adolescents: Effects of an AIDS prevention intervention. *Amer J Public Health*, **82**: 372-377.

Ku, L., Sonenstein, F.L., Pleck, J.H. (1993) Factors Influencing First Intercourse for Teenage Men. *Public Health Reports,* **108:** 680-694.

Levy, S.R., Lampman, C., Handler, A. *et al.,* (1993) Young Adolescent Attitudes toward Sex and Substance Use: Implications for AIDS Prevention. *AIDS Ed and Prev,* **5:** 340-341.

Lui, K, Darrow, W.W., Rutherford, G.W. (1988) A model-based estimate of the mean incubation period for AIDS in homosexual men. *Science,* **240:** 1333-1335.

Mahoney, C.A., Thombs, D.L., Ford, O.J., (1995) Health Belief and Self-Efficacy Modes: Their Utility in Explaining College Student Condom Use. *AIDS Ed and Prev,* **7:** 32-49.

Maticka-Tyndale, E. (1991) Modification of sexual activities in the era of AIDS: A trend analysis of adolescent sexual activities. *Youth & Society,* **23:** 31-49.

Orr, D.P., Beiter, M., & Ingersoll, G. (1991) Premature Sexual Activity as an indicator of psychosocial risk. *Pediatrics,* **87:** 141-147.

Rotheram-Borus, M.J., Mahler, K.A., & Rosario, M. (1995) Aids Prevention with Adolescents. *AIDS Ed and Prev,* 7: 320-336.

St. Louis, M.E., Conway, G.A., Hayman, C.R., *et al.,* (1991) Human Immunodeficiency Virus Infection in Disadvantaged Adolescents, Findings From the US Job Corps. *Journal American Medical Association,* **260:** 2387-2391.

Skurnick, J.H., Johnson, R.L., Quinones, M.A., Louria, D.B. (1991) New Jersey High School Students' Knowledge, Attitudes and Behavior Regarding AIDS. *AIDS Education and Prevention,* **3:** 21-30.

Stanton, B., Xiaoming, L., Black, M., *et al.* (1994) Sexual Practices and Intentions Among Preadolescent and Early Adolescent Low-Income Urban African-Americans. *Pediatrics,* **93:** 966-973.

Statistical Abstract of the United States. (1992) *The National Data Book (112th Ed.).* Washington, D.C.: United States Department of Commerce, Economics and Statistics Administration, Bureau of the Census.

Stiffman, A.R., Earls, F., Dore, P. (1992) Changes in acquired immunodeficiency syndrome-related risk behavior after adolescence: Relationship to knowledge and experience concerning human immunodeficiency virus infection. *Pediatrics,* **89:** 950-955.

Vermund, S.H., Hein, K., Gayle, H.D., *et al.* (1989) Acquired Immune Deficiency Syndrome Among Adolescents. *Amer J of Diseases of Children,* **143:** 1220-1225.

Walter, H.J., Vaughn, R.D., Cohall, A.T. (1991) Psychological influences on acquired immune deficiency syndrome-Risk behaviors among high school students. *Pediatrics,* **88:** 846-852.

Warden, M.A., Koballa, T.R., (1995) Using Students' Salient Beliefs to Design an Instructional Intervention to Promote AIDS Compassion and Understanding in the Middle School. *AIDS Ed. and Prev,* 7: 60-73.

Weisse, C.S., Turbiasz, A.A., Whitney, D.J., (1995) Behavioral Training and AIDS Risk Reduction: Overcoming Barriers to Condom Use. *AIDS Ed and Prev,* **7:** 50-59.

5

Facts and Fictions of Adolescent Risk

SUSAN KIPPAX & JUNE CRAWFORD

INTRODUCTION

This chapter takes issue with a number of assumptions: assumptions that are often made with regard to adolescents' risk of HIV infection. It interrogates a number of concepts including 'adolescent' and 'vulnerability' and problematises the relationship between youth and risk-taking.

Since the beginning of the HIV epidemic, there have been many studies of adolescents generally focusing on heterosexual samples. In many of these studies it is common to find adolescents positioned as risk-takers (e.g. Strunin & Hingson, 1987; Greig & Raphael, 1989; Trad, 1994). Risk taking is, in turn, accounted for in terms of stereotypical thinking (Boyer & Kegeles, 1991); developmental limitations in cognitive and social abilities (Brooks-Gunn, Boyer & Hein, 1988) and tendencies to conformity (King *et al.*, 1989). It is thus often assumed, despite evidence to the contrary, that young people, especially adolescents, are especially vulnerable to HIV.

When HIV surveillance figures for young and old are compared, and where data are available to compare the sexual practices of young and old, adolescents and those under twenty five are revealed to be no more at risk of HIV infection that those aged twenty years and older. This chapter describes these figures and studies.

Our analysis indicates that it is not age per see which places one at greater risk of HIV. Rather, the important predictors of risk are cultural, social and contextual. Social and cultural disadvantage, for example, may place young people at risk, but social and cultural factors of disadvantage are not 'natural' to youth nor are they immanent characteristics of the young.

SOME DEFINITIONS

As Ridge, Plummer & Minichiello (1994) have noted, studies focusing on adolescents or 'youth' typically ignore gay and bisexual men. In this chapter we define 'adolescent' to mean people, including those homosexually active, aged under twenty years, we define 'young' to refer to those aged under twenty five years and we use the term 'older' to refer to those twenty five years and older.

The transmission of HIV infection requires two conditions:

★ engaging in a behaviour that is likely to lead to HIV infection, and in the context of this chapter we focus on one set of such risky practices, namely unprotected sexual intercourse (vaginal, anal or oral-genital); and

★ engaging in one of the above behaviours with an HIV-infected person.

Thus, in the context of HIV, 'risk' has two meanings. One meaning is associated with the behaviour which places one or one's sexual partner at risk. The behaviour is a risk behaviour because of the likelihood of virus transmission from one person to another: for example, both anal and vaginal intercourse are risk behaviours while masturbation is not. The other meaning is associated with the probability of engaging in such a risk behaviour with an HIV infected person. This 'risk' is related to the prevalence of HIV in the population and is thereby also associated with number of sexual partners: in a population with a high prevalence of HIV, a person's risk of HIV increases in terms of number of sexual partners.

The primary focus of this chapter is on behaviour-related risks and, in this chapter behaviour-related risks are measured with reference to frequency of anal and vaginal intercourse with casual as well as regular sexual partners, frequency of condom use and, in regard to the high prevalence population of homosexually active men, number of casual sexual partners.

The first section of this chapter is focused on whether or not adolescents are more or less at risk of HIV than other sections of the population. Two empirical questions are addressed:

(1) is HIV more prevalent in the adolescent population; and

(2) do adolescents and young people engage in more or less risk-related behaviour than older people?

These two questions are addressed with reference to findings which are, in the main, derived from current Australian studies. Restricting these data to Australia and to populations with broadly similar socio-economic backgrounds overcomes the problem of confounding age with cultural and social factors. It must be borne in mind that in Australia over 85% of HIV positive diagnoses are among gay and bisexual men.

EPIDEMIOLOGY OF HIV

The data examined here derive from Australian surveillance data (Australian HIV Surveillance Report, 1994) and from on ongoing study of recent seroconverters among homosexually active men in Australia (Kippax *et al.*, 1994).

INCIDENCE AND PREVALENCE

In Australia, data from the National Centre in Epidemiology and Clinical Research with respect to HIV diagnoses reveal no evidence that young age in associated with increased incidence of HIV infection. Table 1 shows the number of HIV positive diagnoses in each age group of sexual and/or IVDU transmission over the years from 1989 to 1994. The number of diagnoses among 13-19 year olds is very small, and, in each of the six years, there is an increasing number of positive diagnoses with increasing age. In addition, there is a marked and steady decrease over time in the number of diagnoses in each age group.

The consistent decreasing number of diagnoses in each age group over time suggests that the difference in number of diagnoses is not solely due to differences in patterns of testing. If the low number of adolescent diagnoses were solely due to different patterns of testing among adolescents, then decreases over time would be different in the different age groups.

Further data are available with respect to diagnosis of AIDS (as opposed to HIV). The Australian HIV Surveillance Report (1994) shows that the diagnosis of AIDS in Australia has occurred and continues to occur most frequently in the 30-39 year age group (40.8%) followed by the 40-49 year age group (28.1%). These figures support the view that there is no 'hidden' epidemic of HIV infection among adolescents.

This view is further supported by 1994 figures on recent seroconverters (those where a previous negative HIV test is available or where there is a well documented seroconversion illness). These figures show that 2% of recent seroconversions fell

Table 1
Number of HIV positive Diagnoses for Sexual and IVDU Transmission Categories by Age Group, 1989 - 1994.

	AGE GROUP				
YEAR	13-19	20-24	25-29	>30	Total
1989	34	201	340	1010	1585
1990	40	199	341	849	1389
1991	22	175	308	896	1401
1992	18	128	252	788	1186
1993	15	141	224	659	1039
1994	19	103	205	564	891

into the 13-19 age group, 53% in the 20-29 age group (with just under two thirds of these falling in the 25-29 year age group), 31% in the 30 to 39 year age group, 10% in the 40-49 age group and the remaining 3% among those older than 40. (Australian HIV Surveillance Report, 1994).

PREDICTORS OR SEROCONVERSION

A study of recent seroconverters (Kippax *et al.*, 1994) found a number of factors were associated with seroconversion. When homosexually active men who had recently seroconverted (men who had had a negative Elisa test followed by a positive Elisa within a 12 month period prior to interview) were compared with controls (men who had had two negative tests in the same time period), men under 35 years of age were twice as likely as men over 35 years of age to have seroconverted. In line with the above surveillance data, however, the mean age of seroconversion in this sample of men was 32 years compared with a mean age of 37 years for the men who had not seroconverted.

In summary, these data demonstrate that adolescents are no more at risk of HIV than those who are older. Indeed these findings indicate that HIV risk increases up to the late twenties and early thirties and then declines.

Epidemiology of Practice

A number of the Australian studies provide information on age-related risk behaviour among homosexually active men and heterosexually active young people. Data describing the sexual practices of homosexually active men in Australia derive from: the Male Call Project, a national survey of homosexually active men, which was carried out in 1992 (Kippax *et al.*, 1994); a Sydney-based cohort study, Sydney Men and Sexual Health, which began recruiting men in 1993 (Prestage *et al.*, 1995); and a Melbourne study which recruited 284 homosexually active men from a number of locations including gay bars and venues and medical and health clinics (Ridge, Plummer & Minichiello, 1994).

The heterosexual data come from two studies; a 1992 national survey of school students (Dunne *et al.*, 1993) and a Sydney-based study of university students which has been collecting data on the sexual practices of first year students since 1988 (Crawford *et al.*, 1990; Crawford *et al.*, 1994; Rodden *et al.*, 1996).

Thus the data examined in this section derive from Australia and were collected between the years 1992 and 1994.

HOMOSEXUALLY ACTIVE MEN

The Male Call Project surveyed a large national sample of homosexually active men, n = 2,583. One hundred and eight of these men were adolescents, that is aged under

Table 2
Percent of Homosexually active men using condoms for regular and casual sex by age group[a]

CONDOM USE
REGULAR PARTNER/S

	MALE CALL				SMASH			
	Under 20	20-24	25-29	30+	Under 20	20-24	25-29	30+
Insertive**						Insertive		
	(n=22)	(n=111)	(n=138)	(n=372)	(n=7)	(n=53)	(n=74)	(n=162)
Always	77.3	59.5	55.8	47.8	57.1	54.7	51.4	48.1
Sometimes	9.1	14.4	12.3	11.0	28.6	15.1	14.9	12.3
Never	13.6	26.1	31.9	41.1	14.3	30.2	33.8	39.5
Receptive*						Receptive		
	(n=25)	(n=121)	(n=125)	(n=353)	(n=8)	(n=58)	(n=67)	(n=149)
Always	72.0	52.1	58.4	46.2	37.5	55.2	43.3	47.0
Sometimes	12.0	12.4	9.6	12.2	25.0	13.8	20.9	9.4
Never	16.0	35.5	32.0	41.5	37.5	31.0	35.8	43.6

CONDOM USE
CASUAL PARTNER/S

	MALE CALL				SMASH			
	Under 20	20-24	25-29	30+	Under 20	20-24	25-29	30+
Insertive***						Insertive		
	(n=43)	(n=115)	(n=184)	(n=468)	(n=7)	(n=58)	(n=83)	(n=188)
Always	74.4	79.1	84.2	79.3	85.7	86.2	86.7	79.8
Sometimes	23.3	14.8	10.9	9.6	14.3	10.3	8.4	11.7
Never	2.3	6.1	4.9	11.1	-	3.4	4.8	8.5
Receptive						Receptive		
	(n=46)	(n=118)	(n=143)	(n=384)	(n=12)	(n=43)	(n=59)	(n=168)
Always	84.8	78.8	82.5	81.3	75.0	86.0	79.7	85.1
Sometimes	13.0	15.3	10.5	8.9	8.3	14.0	16.9	9.5
Never	2.2	5.9	7.0	9.9	16.7	-	3.4	5.4

[a] Only men engaging in anal intercourse with a casual and/or regular partner are included

* $p < 0.10$ ** $p < 0.05$ *** $p < 0.005$

20 years, 421 were young, that is, aged between 20 and 24, and a further 512 were aged between 25 and 29 years.

Young men are more likely to be in monogamous relationships than older men. Three were, however, no age-related differences with regard to number of sexual partners as these young men were less likely to be in regular or committed relationships in which casual sexual relations were accepted and just as likely as older men to be in casual sex only relationships. The same young men were sexually more active than older men. Adolescent men were more likely to have sex more frequently with their regular sexual partners than men of any other age, but there were no age differences with respect to frequency of sex with casual partners.

The younger men in the sample, particularly those aged between 20 and 24, engaged significantly more often in receptive anal intercourse with their regular and casual partners than men older than themselves but there were no age-related differences with regard to insertive anal intercourse.

The greater likelihood of receptive anal intercourse and the greater sexual activity place these young and adolescent men at risk. These men, particularly the adolescent men, however, were more likely to have used condoms consistently in the last six months for insertive and receptive anal intercourse with their regular partners and there were few age-related differences in condom use with causal partners (see Table 2). These same men were also more likely to favour condoms than those aged 30 years and over and were less likely to have experienced difficulties (breakage or slippage) when using them.

Findings from the Sydney Men and Sexual Health study (Prestage *et al.*, 1995), confirm that adolescent and young homosexually active men who took part in the study in 1993/4 are no more at risk of HIV infection than their older counterparts with reference to unprotected anal intercourse (see Table 2). The adolescent and young men were more likely to have engaged in receptive anal intercourse with both their regular and casual partners than their older counterparts but were no more or less likely to have used condoms in the last six months with both their regular and casual partners than their older counterparts. There were no age-related differences with regard to number of sexual partners.

The data from the Melbourne study confirm the above. Although Ridge, Plummer, Minichiello (1994) did not distinguish regular from casual partners or insertive from receptive anal intercourse, there were no age-related differences between the men in regard to anal intercourse. Between 63 and 85% of the men reported no unprotected anal sex in the three month period prior to interview.

These three sets of behavioural data match the surveillance data. Adolescent men and young men aged under twenty five do not appear to be more at risk of HIV than men aged twenty five and older at least as far as behaviour-related risk is concerned. There is some cause for concern with regard to the slightly higher likelihood of adolescent men being the receptive partner in casual sexual encounters, a point to which we shall return later in the chapter. Further, if the age-related HIV prevalence data are also taken into account, adolescent and young men in Australia whose sexual partners are aged between twenty five and thirty five years, are somewhat more at risk than those whose sexual partners are closer to their own age.

HETEROSEXUAL STUDENTS

The national high school student survey collected data from students in Year 10 (mean age 15 years, 4 months) Year 11 (mean age 16 years and 6 months) and Year 12 (mean age 17 years and 7 months) with regard to number of sexual partners and

Table 3
Percent of Heterosexually active school students using condoms by school year, 1992

CONDOM USE	MALE SCHOOL STUDENTS			FEMALE SCHOOL STUDENTS		
	Year 10 (n=108)	11 (n=132)	12 (n=174)	Year 10 (n=105)	11 (n=197)	12 (n=225)
Always	60.3	53.9	53.6	39.8	41.9	27.7
Often	12.5	11.2	18.4	24.3	18.1	29.2
Sometimes	15.6	23.8	14.4	20.5	24.1	26.8
Never	11.6	11.1	13.6	15.4	15.9	16.2

frequency of condom use in the year prior to interview (n = 2,656). Data were also obtained from the same students with regard to last sexual encounter.

Between 21% of students in Year 10 and 49% of students in Year 12 reported that they had engaged in sex and of these sexually experienced students, approximately half of the male students reported that they had more than one sexual partner, while around 40% of the female students reported having had sex with more than one partner. A majority of the sexually experienced students reported condom use at least some of the time (see Table 3).

These data indicate a reasonably high rate for condom use. The data on condom use during the most recent intercourse confirm this picture: 71.6% of the male students and 53.4% of the female students reported condom use during the most recent intercourse.

Although data have been collected since 1988 from tertiary students as they enter a university in Sydney, the data presented here refer only to the 1992 data. Although approximately only 50% of the 18 and 19 year old students are sexually experienced when they enter university, most of those over twenty are sexually experienced. There were differences between the male and female students with respect to the number of sexual partners which increases with age.

When the data on the condom use of school students, aged between 14 and 18 years, are compared with data for tertiary students attending a university in Sydney, an interesting trend emerges. The younger the student, the more likely that condoms are used (see Table 4). These significant age-related differences hold for both male and female students.

Data from a recently completed study of university students in Melbourne, Australia confirm the above picture. (Rosenthal, *et al.*, 1996). Of those sampled in 1994, most of whom were aged 18 to 19 years, 58.5% of the female students and 69% of the male students reported always using condoms for vaginal sex with their casual partners. The figures were somewhat lower for regular partners (42.7% and 50% respectively).

In general, the findings on heterosexual and homosexual risk practices show that adolescents and young men and women engage in sexual practices that are no more risky than those of older age groups. There is some indication that their practice is safer, at least with regard to condom use. This is particularly true of young heterosexuals. It is also notable that homosexually active young people behave more safely than young heterosexuals. Given the epidemiology of HIV this is not surprising.

One possible interpretation of these data is that condoms have become part of the taken-for-granted reality of many young people's lives, as well as and especially among those who are homosexually active. These findings confirm earlier findings that HIV education and prevention campaigns, in general, are associated with the up-take of preventive behaviour (Wight, 1992; Grunseit *et al.*, in press). There are generational as well as developmental changes occurring with regard to safe sexual practice.

Risk of HIV among the Young

As these findings do not support the view that the young are comparatively more at risk of HIV, why is there what appears to be an exaggerated concern for them? It is not that the Australian data are an exception.

In the United States, surveillance data tell a similar if somewhat more complex story. Kipke, Futterman and Hein (1990) reported that surveillance data obtained from military recruits in New York State showed a seroprevalence rate of 3.0 per 1,000 for those under twenty one years of age compared with a rate of 10.3 per 1,000 for all age groups. These data show that in these populations the young are only one-third as likely to be HIV positive as those in older age groups.

Table 4
Percent of heterosexually active university students using condoms for regular and casual sex by age, 1992[a]

CONDOM USE REGULAR PARTNER/S	Male University Students			Female University Students		
	Under 20 (n=68)	20-24 (n=63)	25+ (n=34)	Under 20 (n=177)	20-24 (n=77)	25+ (n=120)
Always	51.5	20.6	11.8	40.1	26.0	13.3
Sometimes	41.2	61.9	76.5	52.5	67.5	61.7
Never	7.4	17.5	11.8	7.3	6.5	25.0
CONDOM USE CASUAL PARTNER/S	Male University Students			Female University Students		
	Under 20 (n=68)	20-24 (n=63)	25+ (n=34)	Under 20 (n=177)	20-24 (n=77)	25+ (n=120)
Always	67.7	35.3	20.6	58.6	42.2	26.5
Sometimes	22.6	52.9	73.5	31.4	51.1	48.5
Never	9.7	11.8	5.9	10.0	6.7	25.0

[a] Only students engaging in sexual intercourse with a casual and/or regular partner are included.

In a separate national sample of job corps applicants, seroprevalence rates per, 1,000 for those in the 16-21 year age group were 7.0 for black young people, 2.4 for hispanic and 1.4 for white. What these data suggest is that social disadvantage (in this case marked by ethnicity) is a strong predictor of seroprevalence among the young.

Findings from studies other than in Australia with regard to age-related risk behaviour are inconsistent. For example, Davies *et al.* (1992 p270) report that among young (under 21 years old) gay men condom use is "marginally more widespread and consistent than among older men", and Buchbinder *et al.* (1994) reporting on a prospective study of homosexually active men from San Francisco, Chicago, and Denver found that age was not predictive of seroconversion.

On the other hand, a study of gay youth in Canada (Myers *et al.,* 1992) and studies of gay youth (under 30 years of age) in San Francisco (Stall *et al.,* 1992) and Amsterdam (van Griensven *et al.,* 1994) found that gay youth were more at risk of HIV than their older counterparts. It is important to note, however, how youth was defined in these latter studies; that is, as under 30 years.

With regard to heterosexual behaviour, findings of studies in the United Kingdom support the findings described above. In the recent national survey of sexual practice (Wellings *et al.,* 1994), condom use among 16-24 year olds was shown, for both men and women, to be higher than for any other age group. In a view of surveys of the sexual behaviour of young people aged between 16 and 24 years, Fife-Schaw and Breakwell (1992) found that condom use declined with age. They surmise (p.197) that the lower usage reported by older sexually active respondents "presumably reflects the higher proportion of them who will have formed stable monogamous relationships". Their summary of findings also indicates that the later the year of the survey, the more likely it was that respondents reported condom use at their most recent sexual intercourse, with 65.7% of male and 50.3% of female 16 to 17 year olds reporting condom use in 1992. In other words, these findings support the view that the up-take of condoms is related to developmental as well as to generational changes. The United Kingdom trends mirror the Australian trends, although it is not possible to compare directly the proportion of adolescents reporting condom use as different questions were asked of the respondents.

Studies in countries other than the United Kingdom and Australia comparing adolescents with older heterosexuals with regard to risk behaviours are hard to find. We have been unable to find any that support the view that adolescent heterosexuals are more at risk or engage in more risky behaviour than those aged 20 years and over. It appears, as noted in the introduction to this chapter, that many researchers simply begin with the assumption that adolescents are peculiarly at risk.

Correlates of HIV Risk

Some researches, for example, Boyer and Kegeles (1991), aware of the paucity of data on age-related HIV figures or related risk behaviours, turn to STD rates and report and "it is estimated that over 60% of the STD cases reported yearly are individuals under the age of 24" (p.12). In Australia, too, Rosenthal and Reichler

(1994) note that STD surveillance in Victoria indicates that adolescents and those under 25 years represent a significant proportion of those with notified STDs while a statewide study of genital chlamydial infection in South Australia revealed that the highest rates of infection occurred among 15 to 19 years olds, both male and female.

Clearly here there is some evidence of adolescent vulnerability with regard to risk of STDs, the data with regard to HIV risk, however, indicate that there may not be a simple and direct relationship between the two. It is important to interrogate the concept 'adolescence' and concepts closely associated with it. It is age that makes one vulnerable to STDs or HIV? When the findings from the above and other studies are examined more closely, it is evident that factors, particularly social and cultural factors, have led to a somewhat misleading view of age as naturally associated with risk.

ETHNICITY

There are suggestions in the findings of the studies reported above the social disadvantage is associated with increased risk of HIV. As noted above, Kipke, Futterman, and Hein (1990) report differences in HIV infection among African, Hispanic and White Americans. Such differences has been noted by others, for example, Millstein (1990) in her analysis of 1990 data on adolescent risk from Centers for Disease Control. DiClemente (1991) likewise reports higher risk among racial and ethnic minority groups in the United States of America. His study focuses on those already socially disadvantaged, namely, incarcerated youth.

With regard to two cross-sectional surveys of homosexually active young men in San Francisco, van Griensven, Koblin and Osmond (1994) report that HIV prevalence was significantly higher among African Americans (21%) than Latinos (10%), Whites (8%) and Asians (4%).

HOMELESSNESS

Millstein (1990) notes higher HIV prevalence among homeless adolescents in the United States. A similar pattern is noted for homosexually active youths. With reference to runaway and homeless adolescents in New York, van Griensven, Koblin and Osmond (1994) note the very high rate of HIV infection among homosexual and bisexual men who were not injecting drug users; 25% tested HIV positive.

Although not strictly related to homelessness, Abrams *et al.* (1992) report on a study of Scottish teenagers. The findings indicate that adolescents who remain at school are more likely to consider condom use with new partners than early school leavers.

In Australia, a number of studies focused on adolescents have found a relationship between homelessness and increased HIV risk behaviours, for example, in Brisbane (Matthews *et al.*, 1990), in Sydney (Howard, 1992) and in Melbourne (Rosenthal, Moore & Bozwell, 1994).

Table 5
Percent of Heterosexually active Unemployed youth using condoms for regular and casual vaginal intercourse by living conditions, 1992[a]

CONDOM USE	HOMELESS		REFUSE		HOME-BASED	
	Casual (n=35)	Regular (n=37)	Casual (n=40	Regular (n=46)	Casual (n=81)	Regular (n=91)
Always	31.4	24.3	42.5	34.8	48.2	34.1
Sometimes	51.4	45.8	42.5	45.6	28.4	39.5
Never	17.1	29.7	15.0	19.6	23.4	26.4

[a] Only those engaging in sexual intercourse with a casual and/or regular partner are included.

An interesting study comparing homelessness, refuge-based and home-based unemployed youth, aged between 14 and 23 years old, report no significant differences between the groups with regard to condom use (Turtle *et al.*, 1994) (see Table 5). Turtle *et al.* (1994) found that approximately 80% of these unemployed youth in Sydney used condoms at least some of the time for vaginal intercourse with a casual sexual partner, while a lower percentage used them for vaginal intercourse with their regular partner/s (see Table 5). When these findings on condom use among Sydney youth in 1992 are compared with the findings for the university students shown in Table 4, it is clear that condom use is higher among the student sample.

Cultural and social disadvantage, as captured in ethnic differences, lack of education and employment and homelessness, appear to have a negative impact on the up-take of safe sexual practices among the young. Young people who are socially disadvantaged and culturally marginalised are clearly more at risk of HIV infection than their more privileged peers.

INTERPERSONAL SKILLS

Sexual experience and identification with particularly well-informed cultural groups may lessen the negative impact of cultural disadvantage. There is evidence from a number of studies that gay community attached homosexually active men in Australia are more likely to have adopted safe sexual practices then men not so attached (Kippax *et al.*, 1993).

Such attachment to community groups not only informs its members about what is safe and unsafe, but imparts confidence that one's sexual partner/s are likely to have the same information. The development of peer norms is important especially with reference to adolescents.

A number of studies have identified particular skills and experience with are likely to be produced within normative boundaries. DiClemente (1991) in the study referred to above notes that young adolescent males who communicate with their sexual partners about HIV are less at risk than their peers who find such talk difficult. Catania *et al.* (1989) similarly found that among adolescent women, greater willingness to talk to their sexual partners about condoms was associated with higher frequency of condom use. Social consensus and emergent cultural norms with regard to condom use, for example, enable such 'talk'. As Romer and Hornik (1992) point out social consensus is vital for the uptake of appropriate behaviour.

In this context, knowledge about HIV transmission is also shared. Adolescents and young people who have been through the education system in recent years (in Australia at least) have high levels of knowledge about the HIV is transmitted. This has been found even among the socially disadvantaged youth of the study by Turtle *et al.* (1994) referred to above. Similarly, young homosexually active men in the Male Call Project (Kippax *et al.*, 1994) were on the whole better informed than those in older age groups. Heterosexual tertiary students are also knowledgeable about HIV transmission, and accuracy of knowledge among students has been shown to increase over the time period from 1990 to 1994 (Rodden *et al.*, 1996).

GENDER AND SEXUAL IDENTITY

As many researchers have pointed out, women are more vulnerable than men and HIV is no exception (see for example, Holland *et al.*, 1992; Kippax *et al.*, 1994). Gender inequality, especially if it is linked with social inequality, may make it difficult for women to negotiate safe sexual practice and to discuss condom use (Crawford *et al.*, 1994).

Women are also at risk because they are the receptive partners in vaginal sex. Being a receptive partner means that one may be positioned, both metaphorically and physically, as passive and weak.

In their study of the sexual behaviour of young gay men in England and Wales, Davies *et al.* (1992) also note that a higher proportion of young gay men engage in receptive anal intercourse. The Australian data reported above with respect to young homosexually active men also hints at the privileging of the insertive sexual partner. Adolescent homosexually active men are more likely than their older peers to engage in receptive anal intercourse, with both their regular and casual sexual partners. As Davies *et al.* (1992, p.270) note, this is not surprising in a culture characterised by an ethos of male superiority juxtaposed alongside a conception of sexual intercourse in terms of penetration and male domination.

CONCLUSION

Empirical data, comparing the 'risk practices' of young and old and the prevention strategies adopted by them, indicate that adolescents are no more at risk of HIV than those who are twenty years of age or older. Only those young people who are culturally, socially or economically disadvantaged appear more likely to engage in unprotected vaginal or anal intercourse than their older counterparts. Risk taking at least with regard to sexual practice does not seem to be a characteristic peculiar to adolescents or the young.

As Warwick and Aggleton (1990) and Aggleton (1992) have argued young people enmasse are not irresponsible, immature, guileless naive, or lacking relevant information. Rather, as far as sexual practice is concerned, they seem as mature, rational, and responsible as those older than themselves.

Given normative changes that seem to have occurred within some cultural and community groups, adolescents' tendency to conformity, if they can be characterised as conformist, may stand them in good stead. Further, given that adolescents have learnt to engage in sexual practice after the advent of HIV/AIDS, they have the advantage of not having to change their sexual behaviour.

It is important not to pathologise adolescence nor to generalise about young people. Doing so may obscure important correlates of risk such as the cultural, social and contextual factors identified in this chapter. Cultural, social and gender inequality place serious constraints on those who lack power to negotiate safe sexual practice. In this regard the young may be vulnerable, particularly when engaging in sex with a partner from an older age group.

This analysis challenges policy to rethink, reconsider and contemplate direction, assumptions and interventions. If the problems of HIV and AIDS in this group are to be properly tackled, alternative explanations and paradigms may need to evolve.

REFERENCES

Abrams, D., Sheeran, P., Abraham, C. and Spears, R. (1992) Context and content: the impact of school-leaving and school-based education on AIDS-relevant cognitions, *AIDS Care*, **4**, 245-258.

Aggleton, P. (1992) Young people, HIV/AIDS and social research, *AIDS Care*, **4**, 243. *Australian HIV Surveillance Report* (1994) National Centre in HIV Epidemiology and Clinical Research, **10**, October.

Brooks-Gunn, J., Boyer, C., Hein, K. (1988) Preventing HIV infection and AIDS in children and adolescents, *American Psychologist*, **43**, 958-964.

Boyer, C., Kegeles, S., (1991) AIDS risk and prevention among adolescents, *Social Science and Medicine*, **33**, 11-23.

Buchbinder, S., Scheer, S., Judson, F., *et al.*, (1994) Predictors of seroconversion in vaccine preparedness studies of gay men, paper presented at *Xth International Conference on AIDS*, (301C), Yokohama, Japan, August.

Catania, J., Coates, J., Greenblatt, R., *et al.* (1989) Predictors of condom use and multiple-partnered sex interventions, *Journal of Sex Research*, **26**, 514-524.

Crawford, J., Turtle, A., & Kippax, S. (1990) Student-favoured strategies for AIDS among sexually active adolescent women: implications for AIDS – related health avoidance, *Australian Journal of Psychology*, **42**, 123-137.

Crawford, J., Kippax S. & Waldby, C. (1994) Women's sex talk and men's sex talk; different worlds, *Feminism and Psychology*, **4**, 571-587.

Crawford, J., Kippax, S. & Rodden, P. (1994) Knowledge and safe sex practice among heterosexual tertiary students as an outcome of sociocultural change, paper presented at the *Xth International AIDS Conference*, Yokohama, Japan, August.

Davies, P., Weatherburn, P., Hunt, A., *et al.* (1992) The sexual behaviour of young gay men in England and Wales, *AIDS Care*, **4**, 259-272.

DiClemente, R., (1991) Predictors of HIV-preventive sexual behaviour in a high-risk adolescent population: the influence of perceived peer norms and sexual communication on incarcerated adolescents' consistent use of condoms, *Journal of Adolescent Health*, **12**, 385-390.

Dunne, M., Donald, M., Lucke, J. *et al.*, (1993) *1992 HIV Risk and Sexual Behaviour Survey in Australian Secondary Schools: Final Report*, Canberra: Australian Government Publishing Service.

Fife-Schaw, C., & Breakwell, G., (1992) Estimating sexual behaviour parameters in the light of AIDS: a review of recent UK studies of young people, *AIDS Care*, **4**, 187-201.

Grieg, R. & Raphael, B. (1989) AIDS prevention and adolescents, *Community Health Studies*, **13**, 211-219.

Grunseit, A., Kippax, S., Aggleton, P., *et al.*, (in press) Sex education and young people's sexual behaviour: a review of studies, *Journal of adolescent research.*

Holland, J., Ramazanoglu, C., Scott, S. *et al.*, (1992) Risk, Power and the possibility of pleasure: young women and safer sex, *AIDS Care*, **4**, 273-283.

Howard, J. (1992) Changes in HIV risk behaviour in Sydney street youth, *Venereology*, **5**, 88-93.

King, A., Beazley, R., Warren, W., *et al.*, J. (1989) *Canada AIDS and Youth Study*, Ottawa, Center for AIDS Health Protection Branch, Health and Welfare, Canada.

Kipke, M., Futterman, D. & Hein, K. (1990) HIV Infection and AIDS during adolescence, *Adolescent Medicine*, **74**, 1149-1167.

Kippax, S., Connell, R. Dowsett, G. & Crawford, J. (1993) *Sustaining Safe Sex: Gay Communities Respond to AIDS*, London: The Falmer Press.

Kippax, S., Crawford, J., & Waldby, C. (1994) Heterosexuality, masculinity and HIV: barriers to safe heterosexual practice, *AIDS*, **8**, (suppl. 1) S315-S323.

Kippax, S., Crawford, J., Rodden, P. & Benton, K. (1994) *Report on Project Male Call*, Canberra: Australian Government Publishing Service.

Kippax, S., Crawford J., Rodden, P. & Noble, J. (1995) Predictors of unprotected anal intercourse with casual partners in a national sample of Australian men, *Australian Journal of Public Health*, **19**, 132-138.

Kippax, S., Kaldor, J., Crofts, N. *et al.* (1994) Risk factors for HIV among homosexually active men, paper presented at the *6th Annual Conference of the Australasian Society for HIV Medicine*, Sydney, November.

Matthews, B., Richardson, K., Price, J. & Williams, G., (1990) Homeless youth and AIDS: knowledge, attitudes and behaviour, *Medical Journal of Australia*, **153**, 20-23.

Millstein, S. (1990) Risk factors for AIDS among adolescents, *New Directions for Child Development*, **50**, 3-15.

Myers, T., Tudiver, F., Kurtz, R., *et al.* (1992) The talking sex project: descriptions of the study population and correlates of sexual practices at baseline, *Canadian Journal of Public Health*, **83**, 47-52.

Prestage, G., Kippax, S., Crawford, J., *et al.* (1995) *A demographic and behavioural profile and young men, 25 and under, in a sample of homosexually active men in Sydney, Australia, Report B.2.* National Centre for HIV Social Research and National Centre in HIV Epidemiology and Clinical Research, Sydney.

Ridge, D., Plummer, D., & Minichiello, V. (1994) Young gay men and HIV: running the risk? *AIDS Care*, **6**, 371-378.

Rodden, P., Crawford, J., Kippax, S. & French, J. (1996) Sexual Practice and understandings of 'Safe Sex.': Assessing change among 18 to 19 year old tertiary students, 1988-1994. *Australian and New Zealand Journal of Public Health*, **20**, 643-648.

Romer, D. & Hornik, R. (1992) HIV education for youth: the importance of social consensus in behaviour change, *AIDS Care*, **4**, 285-303.

Rosenthal, D., Moore, S. & Buzwell, S. (1994) Homeless youths: sexual and drug related behaviour, sexual beliefs, and HIV/AIDS risk, *AIDS Care*, **6**, 83-94.

Rosenthal, D. & Reichler, H. (1994) *Young heterosexuals, HIV/AIDS, and STDs*, Report prepared for the Department of Human Services and Health, Canberra, Australia, September, Centre for the Study of Sexually Transmissible Diseases, La Trobe University.

Rosenthal, D., Smith, A., Reichler, H. & Moore, S. (1996) Changes in university undergraduates' HIV-related knowledge, attitudes and behaviour, 1989-94, *Genitourinary Medicine*, **72**, 123-127.

Stall, R., Barrett, D., Bye, L. *et al.* (1992) A comparison of younger and older gay men's HIV risk-taking behaviours: the communication technologies 1989 cross-sectional survey, *Journal of Acquired Immune Deficiency Syndromes*, **5**, 682-687.

Strunin, L. & Hingson, R. (1987) Acquired immunodeficiency syndrome and adolescents: Knowledge, beliefs and attitudes and behaviours, *Pediatrics*, **79**, 825-828.

Trad, P. (1994) A developmental model for risk avoidance in adolescents confronting AIDS, *AIDS Education and Prevention*, **6**, 322-338.

Turtle, A., Atashkar, I., Bertuch, M. *et al.* (1994) Reactions to HIV/AIDS of unemployed Australian youth in varying living conditions, *Venereology*, 7, 125-129.

van Griensven, G., Page, K., Veugelers, P. *et al.* (1994) Comparing old and young gay men in San Francisco and Amsterdam; substantial decrease in risk behaviour over time, paper presented in *Xth International Conference on AIDS*, (302C), Yokohama, Japan, August.

van Griensven, G., Koblin, B. & Osmond, D. (1994) Risk behaviour and HIV Infection among younger homosexual men, *AIDS*, **8** (suppl 1) S125-S130.

Warwick, I. & Aggleton, P. (1990) 'Adolescents', young people and AIDS research, in P. Aggleton, P. Davies and G. Hart (eds.) *AIDS: Individual, Cultural, and Policy Dimensions*, 89-102. London: The Falmer Press.

Wellings, K. Field, J., Johnson, A. & Wadsworth, J. (1994) *Sexual Behaviour in Britain: The National Survey of Sexual Attitudes and Lifestyles*, London: Penguin Books.

Wight, D. (1992) Impediments to safer heterosexual sex: a review of research with young people, *AIDS Care*, **4**, 11-21.

6

Young People, Sexuality, and HIV and AIDS Education

PETER AGGLETON & IAN WARWICK

INTRODUCTION

'Adolescence is a time of growth and experimentation, a period marked by establishing autonomy and confronting new challenges. It is also a period in which many adolescents will initiate sexual and drug-related risk behaviours that increase the probability of HIV infection. (DiClemente, 1992:xi)

'Adolescents are particularly at risk of STDs because of their high levels of sexual activity, sexual experimentation, often with multiple partner, and their failure to use condoms consistently, or even at all.' (Moore & Rosenthal, 1994: 18)

'Adolescence is the transitional phase between childhood and adulthood, characterised by experimentation and rapid change (...) Passing through the inter-related stages of cognitive, social, emotional and physical development of adolescence requires considerable adaptation, and failure to negotiate these developmental hurdles successfully may have far-reaching consequences.' (Department of Health, 1994:74)

YOUNG PEOPLE AND AIDS

Some six years ago, while reviewing the published literature on young people on AIDS, we described the narrow and stereotypical ways in which young people have been portrayed in relation in the epidemic (Warwick & Aggleton, 1990). Central among the images then to be found in the literature were those of the 'unknowledgeable adolescent', the 'high risk adolescent', the 'over-determined adolescent' and the 'tragic adolescent'. The first of these categories by far the most dominant at the time, suggested that young people were largely ignorant of the threat posed by HIV disease and of the means whereby to prevent infection (see for example, DiClemente, Zorn & Temoshok, 1986). The second linked more closely to beliefs that young people, of their essence, are more prone to risk-taking than adults, and derived in all likelihood from the 'thrills, pills and spills' theory of youth promulgated, both then and now, by popular psychology and the mass media (see, for example, Strunin & Hingson, 1987). The third characterisation, which combines both biological and social determinisms, suggests that young people's behaviour is largely the product of forces beyond their control: forces which propel them towards conformity with peer group norms and the need to be part of a group (see, for example, King *et al.,* 1989). The fourth image was reserved for those young people unfortunate enough to have developed AIDS, and for whom the supposed 'innocence' of youth was at contradiction with the events that had come to pass (see, for example, Wishon, 1988.)

It is sad to say that in the ensuing years such images have continued to predominate in academic accounts of young people and AIDS, coming to constitute the taken-for-granted commonsense of much of the international research community, most especially those working in the fields of psychology and behavioural medicine. A recent article in the journal *AIDS Education and Prevention,* for example, contained that claim that 'adolescents have developmental capabilities that may serve to limit their understanding of the consequences of their actions and put them at greater risk for inadvertent exposure to HIV disease (Newman *et al.,* 19932:328, with emphasis added), whereas another article in this same journal suggested that 'the tendency to underestimate susceptibility may be especially true among adolescents, who characteristically view themselves as invincible (Mickler, 1993:44, with emphasis added).

But several new species have been added to this earlier menagerie of 'adolescent' types. Included among these are the 'unrealistically optimistic' adolescent (Moore & Rosenthal, 1994), the 'unrealistically optimistic' adolescent (Moore & Rosenthal, 1994), the 'slavishly conformist' adolescent (Bowser & Wingood, 1992), the 'know-it-all' adolescent (Stevenson *et al.,* 1995, the adolescent who lacks 'anticipatory awareness' (Rotheram-Borus, Koopmen & Rosario, 1992), the adolescent who relies on 'sexual mythologies and misplaced beliefs' (Rosenthal, Moore & Buzwell, 1994), and the adolescent who is prone to the influence of, and we quote, 'anti-prevention reference group social norms' (Fisher, Misovich & Fisher, 1992). Clearly there exists no shortage of explanations as to why young people may face heightened risks.

Two factors are worthy of particular attention in many of the above accounts. First, they near universally posit the existence of deficits and/or pathology in young people's personal and social functioning. Second, none of them offers an explicitly classed, gendered or culturally differentiated account of young people and their HIV-related needs. Instead, age is held to be *the* determining factor linking together disparate experiences and predicaments. In many ways this is curious given the care now taken in the literature on adults and AIDS to distinguish between gender, social background, ethnicity and, most especially, sexuality, in determining HIV-related risk. It is, however, indicative of the extent to which popular ideologies of adolescence seem literally to have won the hearts and *minds* of those working in the field.

Few approaches engage either with young people's sexual desires, motivations and behaviours in ways that are likely to be meaningful to the individuals concerned. Indeed in perhaps the majority of contemporary accounts, sexuality is not discussed at all, it being assumed that all young people are unequivocally heterosexual; and sexual behaviour is reduced to the effects of biology, poor socialization and faulty learning, boredom and frustration, among other factors. More often than not it is the negative consequences of sexual behaviour that are focused on, such as unwanted teenage pregnancy and the acquisition of sexually transmitted diseases. This emphasis is unfortunate in two respects: not only does it provide a limited understanding of young people and their HIV and AIDS-related needs, it also encourages us to see young people's sexuality in negative terms – as something that needs to be restrained and controlled, not as a creative force capable of offering pleasure, fulfilment and growth.

Definitions of sexual health vary from those that are negative, linking sexual health to the absence of unwanted pregnancy and disease, to those that are more affirmative, emphasising, for example, the 'capacity to enjoy and express sexuality without guilt and shame in fulfilling, emotional relationships' (WHO, 1987). Regardless of the definition adopted, and just like their adult counterparts, young people continue to face a number of threats to their health and well-being, both sexually and reproductively. While the scale of this threat is difficult to determine, and while its determinants remain complex and ill-defined, the problem is not insignificant given that a substantial number of people with AIDS are reported as having acquired HIV infection during their late teens and early twenties. Recent British data, for example, suggests that 48% of 16 years-olds, 61% of 17 year-olds and 78% of 19 year-olds report having had sex with, or having been sexually active with, another person. The most frequently reported form of protection used during sexual intercourse is the contraceptive pill, followed by the condom. But condom use declines rapidly with age. Whereas 77% of sexually active young men aged 16 reported using a condom at last intercourse, only 47% of 19 year-olds report having used one the last time they had sex (Health Education Authority, 1992). Comparable findings emerge from studies conducted elsewhere in the world, although there is evidence from Switzerland that it may be possible to arrest this decline with appropriate health promotion interventions (WHO, 1992).

MEANINGFUL VERSUS RHETORICAL HEALTH PROMOTION

It is central to the argument offered in this chapter that if health promotion related to HIV and AIDS is to be meaningful, it must speak to lived experience. That is, it should engage with what young people believe to be true about their own lives – their concerns and aspirations, and the everyday dilemmas that confront them. This is what we mean when we talk of meaningful health promotion, an activity that must be carefully differentiated from others that may seemingly be concerned with the promotion of health, but which in reality fail to engage with experience as it is actually lived.

In the field of HIV and AIDS, numerous more rhetorical forms of health promotion abound. They include those that talk of the need to return to 'traditional values' of chastity and monogamy in circumstances where historically neither of these practices has characterised sexual life; they include those that suggest that young women should be offered the skills by which to negotiate for safer sex in circumstances where patriarchy and tradition render such 'negotiation' all but impossible; and they include those interventions that speak only to heterosexual desires and practices in circumstances where intercourse between partners of the same sex may be common, even if it is not openly acknowledged or seen as 'real sex'.

Meaningful HIV and AIDS-related health promotion, on the other hand, starts from the recognition that people's experience varies in complex and perhaps contradictory ways, according to their social background, status, gender, sexuality and ethnicity. It thereby prioritizes needs assessment as the first stage in learning about individual's circumstances and needs. More than this, however, it recognizes that human lives are situated – that is, they take place within particular settings and contexts. These environments not only give meaning to what we as people do, they set limits upon what it is possible to do, and how it is possible to live. What counts as sex and legitimate sexual expression, what opportunities there are to express oneself sexually, and what constraints affect the expression of sexual desires – all are dependent upon situation and context (Parker, 1994). In some parts of the world, for example, early sexual experience is proscribed, whereas in others it is encouraged. In some places, sex between those who are young and those who are older is seen as relatively natural, whereas in others it is seen as aberrant. In some contexts, sex between two individuals of the same sex may be seen as nothing unusual, whereas in others it is viewed as abnormal or a 'perversion. In some societies, sex involving the regular exchange of gifts or money is seen as 'prostitution', whereas in others it is seen as a way of showing respect and commitment (Aggleton, 1993).

The idea that context and environment are powerful determinants of health, constraining individuals in their actions and limiting the capacity to 'choose' healthy lifestyles, is central to much of what constitutes good practice in health promotion. It finds expression in the Ottawa Charter (WHO, 1986) among other international declarations, which emphasizes the political, economic and social factors affecting health and well-being, and which focuses attention on policy and environment as ways of promoting better health. It has also led to the development of a wide range of health promoting interventions. In the field of HIV and AIDS, for example, it has given new emphasis to what O'Reilly and Piot (in press) have called enabling interventions, and what Sweat and Dimension (1995) have called structural and environmental interventions – styles of health promotion that move beyond persuasion as a way of reducing HIV-related risk, to modify the economic, political and social circumstances in which individuals live their lives. These include economic interventions to reduce the likelihood that parents will sell their daughters and sons into prostitution, and legislation making the use of condoms in brothels mandatory and enforceable by brothel owners and managers.

APPROACHES

Since the start of epidemic, efforts have been made to undertake HIV and AIDS-related health promotion with young people in a variety of settings and in range of ways. Preferred settings include those both in and out of school. Techniques used vary from formal instruction, through skill-based approaches to more participatory and experiential forms of learning, some of which aim to bring about wide reaching social change (Aggleton, 1989). Much advocated in recent years has been peer-led education in which young people themselves undertake HIV and AIDS-related health promotion work. While some approaches have been focused so as to meet the needs of particular groups of young people (e.g. young gay men, young people who inject drugs, young Black people, young homeless people etc.), others have adopted a more generic approach. An important distinction can be drawn between sex positive and sex negative styles of HIV and AIDS-related health promotion. Whereas the former tend to promote sex as an enriching and fulfilling aspect of human behaviour, and most generally aim to make sex safer, the latter see sexual desires and sexual expression more negatively, as motivations and behaviours that need to be controlled and/or reserved for expression only in special occasions and contexts (e.g. within marriage).

Regardless of the approach adopted, a number of common principles have been identified underpinning those forms of HIV and AIDS-related health promotion that are most likely to prove effective in bringing about desired objectives. These include: the provision of relevant information, activities to encourage personal appraisal of risk, training in skills for sexual negotiation and the use of condoms, and access to resources such as condoms and appropriate health services (Aggleton, 1996). It follows therefore that initiatives with young people in school or out of school constitute but one element in the overall package of intervention necessary to promote and maintain, HIV-related risk reduction. Recognising this is the first step towards having realistic expectations about what a particular initiative with young people can and can not achieve.

School-based approaches

Since early in the epidemic, schools have been seen as important environments in which to undertake work with young people on HIV and AIDS. One reason for this is that they are one of the few contexts in which it is possible to encounter relatively large numbers of young people together – they offer the potential at least for mass education on a scale that is elsewhere difficult. But they are also hierarchical institutions in which relations of power, between teachers and pupils as well as between pupils themselves, come into play. Because of this they may be more suited to certain forms of HIV and AIDS-related health promotion than others, most notably those that adopt a relatively didactic and formal approach. This is not to argue, however, that more open-ended, exploratory and participatory kinds of education cannot be made to work in such environments, they can. But teachers and pupils require adequate preparation for this kind of work, particularly if it is likely to involve encountering and perhaps re-evaluating personal feelings about sex, sexuality and sexual expression.

School-based approaches to HIV and AIDS-related education vary widely both in their goals and in the educational strategies that are used to bring these about. While information-based approaches have been widely used, involving talks, lectures, guest speakers and videos, we should not imagine that they are capable of doing much other than bringing about changes in knowledge. The modification of attitudes and behaviours requires the more active involvement of learners, and encourages the use of more participatory approaches such as games, role plays, simulations and skills training. But even here we should guard against a tendency to imagine that skills acquired in one setting are necessarily transferable to other environments. It is not inconceivable for young people to perform well when practising sexual negotiation and condom use skills in the classroom yet to find themselves unable to act in a similar way in real life where the pressures towards unsafe sex may be greater and/or where having unprotected sex is taken as being a signal of commitment and trust. Growing recognition of this fact has led several authors to argue for parallel but complementary intervention in and out of school.

In Britain and in some other countries, there has been much controversy about the best way of delivering HIV and AIDS-related education, with some favouring a topic-based approach, and others arguing for its integration into subjects such as biology and science, themes such as health education, and more general areas of work such as tutoring and personal and social education. Broadly speaking, existing curriculum materials can be divided into five main types – those that adopt an explicit moral position, be it the promotion of certain spiritual or moral values or the challenging of discrimination and stereotypes; those that offer a humanistic and experiential pragmatic approach; those that offer a technicist or skills-based pragmatic approach; those that claim to be based upon psychosocial models of sexual risk taking behaviour; and those that attempt to integrate work on HIV and AIDS within a broader framework for the promotion of sexual health.

While favouring integration as a general principle, the World Health Organisation with UNESCO has recently published a prototype curriculum for schools with a strong participatory emphasis (WHO, 1994). This relatively non-judgemental skill-based curriculum seeks to promote five related sets of skills among young people including those related to risk assessment, sexual negotiation, the practice of safe sexual behaviour, the use of STD and HIV-related services, and the avoidance of sexual violence.

Out of school approaches

Out of school, an important distinction can be drawn between what may be called planned approaches to HIV and AIDS-related health promotion and those that are more adventitious, seizing the opportunity as and when it arises. Perhaps the majority of interventions worldwide have been of the latter kind, as youth workers and youth leaders have acted spontaneously to address HIV and AIDS-relevant concerns when they are expressed by young people, or in response to particular situations, such as the discovery that a friend or relative has HIV disease. Clearly, adults working with young people need to be adequately prepared for such interventions if their responses are to promote understanding, alleviate unnecessary anxieties and enable young people to develop the skills whereby to protect themselves and others against infection. A number of resources have been produced to facilitate this, although their availability and training in their use may be limited.

More structured approaches to the HIV and AIDS-related health promotion with young people in out of school settings frequently involve incorporating a consideration of HIV-related risks, safer sex and safer drug use into some kind of developmental youth work (Smith, 1991). Here, the aim may be to introduce young people in a relatively structured way to issues raised by HIV and AIDS, sexuality, substance use and personal relationships. The success of such approaches depends ultimately both on the skills of the practitioner and on there being a periodicity or continuity of contact between youth workers and youth leader and young people themselves. As a contribution towards such work, the World Health Organisation has produced guidelines and sample exercises for use with young people in out of school contexts (WHO, 1991), and there exist other resources with a similar purpose (e.g. Aggleton *et al.,* 1990).

There has been much discussion in recent years concerning the role of peer-led education in HIV and AIDS-related peer education. This has been triggered by the realisation that young people may be better able to access their peers than adults, by the possibility that for some young people at least peers may be seen as more credible than adults, and by the fact that peer-led education can be a relatively inexpensive way of increasing awareness and perhaps, changing attitudes. But behind the rhetoric about the value of this approach lies much conceptual and methodological confusion (see for example BGA, 1994). Indeed, rather than describing one particular approach to health promotion, the term peer-led education encompasses a range of strategies and techniques. These include peer communication, most usually consisting of one-off information activities; peer counselling, most usually focusing on personal problems and problem solving; and peer education generally involving young people acting as educators, role models, organizers and discussion leaders (Fee & Youssef, 1993). To these can be added peer influence and peer participation as ways of bringing about change in sexual and drug-related behaviour (Kinder, 1995). Several resources to promote the use of peer-led education as part of HIV and AIDS-related health promotion now exist (e.g. Cohen & Fuccillo, 1991; Downes, 1995).

A number of challenges have been identified for those wishing to use peer-led education in their work. They include how best to identify suitable peer leaders, how to provide training and support to such leaders, how to ensure that the messages conveyed are non-discriminatory and non-stigmatizing, how to ensure that peer-led approaches reach a sufficiently large number of young people, and how to ensure that peer-led education is involving and participatory rather than didactic (BGA, 1994).

Focused approaches

Throughout much of the preceding discussion it has been assumed that HIV and AIDS-related health promotion in and out of school is delivered in a way sensitive to the needs of different groups of young people. This requires teachers and youth workers to be aware of varying needs and willing to adapt curriculum and other resources as necessary. However, even the best planned work conducted with heterogeneous or socially diverse groups of young people may fail to meet particular needs unless accompanied by more focused interventions. This is particularly true in relation to young people who are socially marginalised by virtue of factors such as their place of residence, their sexuality, homelessness, and through involvement in illicit drug use.

Young people in rural areas, for example, may have special needs when it comes to HIV and AIDS-related health promotion. Some of these may be linked to general social issues such as lack of employment opportunities perhaps made worse through rural recession. Others may be connected to the non-availability of youth oriented health services and safer sex information, specific understandings of what it is to be a 'man' or a 'woman', and the near impossibility of anonymity when purchasing condoms or using local health services. Additionally, ideologies suggesting that rural areas may be relatively untouched by 'city problems' and that sexual life is characterised by 'clean living' may pose special challenges for HIV and AIDS-related work, especially when such ideologies are at odds with reality in these same settings (Harrison *et al.*, 1995). As yet, relatively few intervention projects have sought to engage with concerns such as these, creating a major challenge for work with young people in the future.

It is increasingly recognised that in many societies young men who have, or would like to have, sex with other men may be particularly vulnerable to HIV infection - through lack of awareness of HIV-related risks, through not having the skills by which to negotiate for safer sex, through their relative powerlessness to insist on safer sex with older partners, among other factors (Sotiropoulos, 1985). While we should take care not to stereotype young gay and bisexual men and their needs, and while there exists debate about the relative risks faced (see, for example, Aggleton, 1995), for a not insignificant number of younger men in the process of coming to recognise that they may not be heterosexual, the risks may be very real.

Meeting the needs of such young men requires specific interventions against the backcloth of wider efforts to promote safer sex among all gay and bisexual men. Such interventions may need to be of several different kinds if they are to meet the needs of a wide range of younger gay and bisexual men. These include specific projects run by HIV and AIDS-related organisations and groups, projects based within youth organisations and youth groups, and activities aiming to attach or link younger gay and bisexual men to the gay community settings in which safer sex has become normative (Knapman, 1995).

Homelessness poses major health challenges for young people, both in advanced industrial societies such as Britain where it is a relatively new phenomenon, and in countries where it has long existed (Luna & Rotheram-Borus, 1992). Not only do homeless young people face enhanced vulnerability as a result of their marginalization from HIV and AIDS-related health promotion activity, they have greater difficulty accessing mainstream health services. They may face additional risks from sex work undertaken for accommodation and money and through injecting drug use (Pennbridge *et al.*, 1992), as well as a result of sexual assault and rape (Bond, Mazin & Jimenez, 1992.)

It has been well documented that HIV-related issues may not rank highly among the concerns of homeless young people. Having something to eat, finding somewhere to live and getting a job can be more pressing demands. HIV and AIDS-related issues must therefore be addressed within a broader context in which attention is given to more general health and social welfare needs, concurrent with HIV-related interventions (Aggleton & Warwick, 1992). A range of successful interventions with homeless young people have been documented, including culturally and gender sensitive programmes that include social skills training and social support (Rotheram-Borus *et al.*, 1991: Warwick & Whitty, 1995).

Since early in the epidemic, young people who inject drugs have been identified as requiring specially focused interventions if they are to be supported in minimizing HIV-related risk. To be successful, such interventions must include components that address injection-related and sexual health needs. A range of health promotion options are needed to address the varying reasons why young people may inject drugs, as well as ways of minimizing harm through the consistent use of clean needles and syringes and through safer sex. Specialist interventions may be needed to meet the needs of young people from minority ethnic communities and/or who have different kinds of involvement with injecting drug use (Crofts, Louie & Rosenthal, 1995).

CONCLUSIONS

Throughout this chapter we have tried to argue for a more realistic and less stereotypical appreciation of young people and HIV and AIDS-related health promotion – one that has its starting point in the patterned diversity of young people's experience and in the variety of needs to which this gives rise. The most effective kinds of HIV and AIDS-related health promotion are therefore likely to have their starting point in local needs assessments conducted with specific groups of young people, rather than in pre-existing 'theories' about adolescence as a stage of life.

In reviewing some of the techniques open to those working with young people, we have drawn attention both to the generic kinds of activities that may be undertaken with relatively heterogeneous groups of young people in and out of school and to the more focused kinds of work needed to complement these broader initiatives. The key to effective work with young people, we would argue, lies in establishing a productive level of complementarity and commensurability between interventions of different kinds, not in searching for one particular solution that 'works'. Because young people's experience varies both temporally and according to circumstances, we should be cautious of trying to identify, by case-control methods or other means, a supposedly universal strategy or means whereby to promote or sustain safer sex. Instead, our concern should be to make available a menu of risk-reduction options and the resources whereby young people can protect themselves and their partners against HIV-related risks. Such as approach calls for both humility and respect on the part of social researchers and health promotion specialists who may be tempted to seek and impose supposedly universal solutions to what are essentially context-specific problems.

REFERENCES

Aplasca, M.R., Siegel, D., Mandel, J., Santana-Arciaga, R.T., Paul, J. *et al.,* (1995) Results of a Model AIDS Prevention Programme for High School Students in the Phillippines. *AIDS 1995,* **9**, S7-S13.

Aggleton, P.J. (1989) Evaluating Health Education about AIDS. In P. Aggleton, G. Hart and P. Davies (Eds.) *AIDS: Social Representations, Social Practices,* Lewes: Falmer Press.

Aggleton, P.J. (1993) Sexual Behaviour Research and AIDS. Plenary Presentation at the AIDS in Africa Conference, Marrakesh.

Aggleton, P.J. (1995) Men who have sex with Men. Social and Behavioural Research: Implications for Needs Assessment. London: Health Education Authority.

Aggleton, P.J. (1996) *Health Promotion and Young People.* London: Institute of Education, Health & Education Research Unit. Report to the Health Education Authority.

Aggleton, P.J., Horsely, C., Wilton, T. & Warwick, I. (1990) AIDS: Working with Young People, Ist Edition, Horsham: AIDS Education and Research Trust.

Aggleton, P.J. Rivers, K. & Warwick, I. (with Horsley C. and Wilton, T.) (1993) *AIDS: Working with Young People, 2nd Edition.* Horsham: AIDS Education and Research Trust.

Aggleton, P. & Warwick, I (Eds) (1992) *Young People, Homelessness and HIV/AIDS.* London: Health Education Authority.

Bond, L., Mazin, R. & Jiminez, M.V. (1992) Street Youth and AIDS. *AIDS Education and Prevention.* Supplement, 14-23.

Bowser, B. & Wingood, G. (1992) Community-based HIV Prevention Programs and Adolescents. In R. DiClemente (ed.) *Adolescents and AIDS,* Newbury Park, CA; Sage.

BGA (1994) Report from the VIth European Consultation on AIDS Prevention Education. Possibilities of Applying Peer Involvement Approaches in HIV Prevention. Koln; Bundeszentrale fur gesundheitliche Aufklarung.

Cohen, B. & Fuccillo, R. (1991) *Peer Leadership Preventing AIDS.* Boston, MA: Medical Foundation.

Crofts, N., Louie, R. & Rosenthal, D. (1995) The First Hit: Initiation into injecting among young people in Melbourne. *National AIDS Bulletin,* **9**, 22-24.

Department of Health (1994) *On the State of the Public Health,* London: HMSO.

DiClemente, R. (Ed.) (1992) *Adolescents and AIDS: a generation in Jeopardy.* Newbury Park, CA: Sage.

DiClemente, R., Zorn, J. and Temoshok, L. (1986) Response by DiClemente *et al., American Journal of Public Health,* 77, 876-877.

Downes, G. (1995) *Peer Education and HIV Prevention.* London: Cultural Partnerships.

Fee, N. & Youssef, M. (1993) Young People, AIDS and STD Prevention: Experiences of Peer Approaches in Developing Countries. Geneva: World Health Organisation, Global Programme on AIDS.

Fisher, J., Misovich, S. & Fisher, W. (1992) Impact of Perceived Social Norms on Adolescents AIDS-Risk Behaviour and Prevention. In R. DiClemente (ed.) *Adolescents and AIDS,* Newbury Park, CA: Sage.

Furnham, A. & Gunter, F. (1988) *The Anatomy of Adolescence.* London: Routledge.

Health Education Authority (1992) *Today's Young Adults.* London: HEA.

Kinder, P. (1995) HIV and AIDS: Looking at Peer Education. *On the Level,* **3**, 41-46.

King, A., Beazley, R., Warren, W., Hankins, C. Robertson, A. et. al (1989) *Canada AIDS and Youth Study.* Ottawa: Center for AIDS Health Promotion Branch, Health and Welfare Canada.

Knapman, R. (1995) The Inside Out Story. *National AIDS Bulletin,* **9**, 26-29.

Luna, G.C. & Rotheram-Borus, M.J. (1992) Street Youth and the AIDS Pandemic. *AIDS Education and Prevention,* Supplement 1, 1-13.

McRobbie, A. (1991) *Feminism and Youth Culture.* Basingstoke: Macmillan.

Mickler, S. (1993) Perceptions of Vulnerability: Impact of AIDS Preventive Behaviour among College Adolescents. *AIDS Education and Prevention,* **5**, 43-53.

Moore, S. & Rosenthal, D. (1994) Youth People Assess their Risk of Sexually Transmissible Diseases. *Psychology and Health,* **10**, 17-31.

Newman, C., Durant, R., Ashworth, C.S. and Gaillard, G. (1993) An Evaluation of a School-based AIDS/HIV Program for Youth Adolescents. *AIDS Education and Prevention,* **5**, 327-339.

O'Reilly K. & Piot, P. (in press) Individual and Community Approaches to STD/HIV Prevention. *Journal of Infectious Diseases* (suppl.)

Parker, R. (1994) Sexual Cultures, HIV Transmission and AIDS Prevention. *AIDS,* **8** (suppl.) S309-14).

Pennbridge, J.N., Freese, T.E. & Mackenzie, R.G. (1992) High-Risk Behaviours among Male Stevenson, H.C., McKee Gay, K. & Josar, L. (1995) Culturally Sensitive AIDS Education and Perceived AIDS Risk Knowledge: Reaching the 'Know it all' Teenager. *AIDS Education and Prevention,* 7, 134-144.

Street Youth in Hollywood, California. *AIDS Education and Prevention,* Supplement, 24-33.

Rosenthal, D., Moore, S. & Buzwell, S. (1994) Homeless Youths: sexual and drug-related behaviour, sexual beliefs and HIV/AIDS risk. *AIDS Care,* **6**, 83-94.

Rotheram-Borus, M., Miller, S., Koopman, C., Haignere, C. & Selfridge, C. (1991) Adolescents Living Safely: *AIDS Awareness, Attitudes, Actions.* New York, NY: HIV Center for Clinical and Behavioural Studies, Colombia University.

Rotheram-Borus, J., Koopman, C. & Rosario, M. (1992) Developmentally Tailoring Prevention Programs: Matching Strategies to Adolescents' Serostatus. In R. DiClemente (ed.) *Adolescents and AIDS.* Newbury Park, CA: Sage.

Smith, M. (1991) Researchers, Practitioners and Work with Young People around HIV/AIDS. In P. Aggleton (Ed.) *Young People and HIV/AIDS,* Swindon; Economic and Social Research Council.

Sotiropoulos, J. (1995) Young People Do Get HIV. *National AIDS Bulletin*, **9**, 10-11.

Strunin, L. and Hingson, P. (1987) Acquired Immunodeficiency Syndrome and Adolescents: Knowledge, Beliefs, Attitudes and Behaviours. *Paediatrics*, **79**, 825-8.

Sweat, M. & Dennison, J. (1995) Reducing HIV Incidence in Developing Countries with Structural Environmental Interventions. *AIDS* (suppl A), **9**, S251-257.

Warwick, I. & Aggleton, P.J. (1990) 'Adolescents', Young People and AIDS Research. In P. Aggleton, P. Davies and G. Hart (Eds.) *AIDS: Individual, Cultural and Policy Dimensions*, Basingstoke, Falmer Press.

Warwick, I. Whitty, G.J. (1995) *When it Matters: Developing HIV and AIDS Education with Young Homeless People*. London: Health Education Authority.

WHO (1986) *Ottawa Charter for Health Promotion*. Ottawa/Geneva; Health and Welfare Canada/World Health Organisation.

WHO (1987) Concepts of Sexual Health, Unpublished Report of a Working Group. Copenhagen: WHO (EURO).

WHO (1994) *Health Education to Prevent AIDS and STD*. Geneva: World Health Organisation/UNESCO.

WHO (1991) *Guide for Developing Health Promotion Projects for AIDS Prevention among Out-of-School Youth*. Geneva, World Health Organisation, Global Programme on AIDS.

WHO (1992) *Effective Approaches to AIDS Prevention: Report of a Meeting, Geneva, 26-29 May*. Geneva, World Health Organisation, Global Programme on AIDS.

Wishon, P. (1988) Children and Youth with AIDS. *International Journal of Adolescence of Youth*, **1**, 213-227.

7

Expanding the Context: Australian Adolescents' Behaviours and Beliefs about HIV/AIDS and other STDs.

DOREEN ROSENTHAL

INTRODUCTION

There has been in Australia, as in other Western countries, increasing attention paid to the sexual practices and HIV/AIDS risk of young people. In Australia, male homosexual/bisexual contact is still overwhelmingly the major risk for HIV/AIDS and present data indicate that the risk of HIV infection for young heterosexuals aged 16 to 24 is low. If, however, the epidemiology of other STDs is considered, the picture is quite different.

While it is difficult to obtain accurate epidemiological data for STDs other than HIV, young people between the ages of 16 and 24 appear to be at high risk compared with those who are older or younger (Stevenson *et al.,* 1992). Data from the United States have shown that the highest rates of chlamydia and gonorrhoea occur among 15 to 19 year-olds. In some populations, such as street youth, rates are as high as 40 to 50 percent. Short (1993) claims that "nearly 25% of all cases of sexually transmitted disease occur in adolescents, with 2.5 million new cases a year, or 1 in 7 of all 15 to 19 year-olds." (p.7). The picture is substantially the same in Australia, with young people representing a significant proportion of those with notified STDs (Hart, 1993; Garland, Gertig, & Mclnnes, 1993; Kovacs, Westcott, Rusden *et al.,* (1987).

Clearly young people are at substantially higher risk of these STDs than they are of being infected with HIV. For example, Donovan (1992) estimates that they have a 500-fold greater risk of contracting chlamydia than of becoming infected with

HIV. There are at least two different and serious consequences of infection with STDs (other than HIV). First, although most are treatable, they can have distressing and debilitating long-term sequelae. For example, chlamydia may result in pelvic inflammatory disease which in turn is a common cause of infertility in women , and genital warts have been linked with increased risk of cervical cancer. Second, the presence of other STDs increases the risk of HIV infection (by one estimate, three to five-fold, Wasserheit, (1992). Moreover, HIV infection appears to increase the prevalence of some STDs. As Short (1993) notes: "Since these STDs in turn also increases the incidence of HIV infection, we have a true `epidemiological synergy', with each infection exacerbating the other" (p.2.) For these reasons, and given that protection against STDs will also provide protection against HIV infection, it is important that the focus of prevention research extends beyond HIV/AIDS to include those other STDs which are more likely to impact on the lives of heterosexual young people.

SEXUAL PRACTICES

According to recent studies in a number of Western countries, the incidence of sexual intercourse is on the increase and the age of first sexual experience is decreasing, especially for girls (Brooks-Gunn & Furstenberg, 1989; Goldman & Goldman, 1988; Hein, 1989, Hofferth & Hayes, 1987; Rollins, 1989). In Australia, non-virgin status is normative by the end of high school (Dunne *et al.,* 1993; Rosenthal, Moore, & Brumen, 1990), and sexual activity begins early for some. For example, 10% of young people in Dunne *et al.,'s* national survey reported having sex by age 13. Levels of sexual activity, are, generally speaking, low, with most young people reporting only one partner and/or infrequent sexual experiences of sex. However, homeless young people, injecting drug users, and those who are unemployed report high levels of sexual activity and risky practices Dunne, Donald, Lucke and Raphael, in press; Loxley & Ovenden, 1992; Rosenthal, Moore, & Buzwell, 1994).

Sexual practices vary, with oral sex being practised by most young people at this age. The incidence of anal sex, while relatively low, occurs with more frequency among some groups and more often with regular than with casual partners (Rosenthal *et al.,* 1990; Turtle *et al.,* 1989). For example, Rosenthal *et al.* (1994) found that 25% of 16 year-old homeless girls and boys reported that they engaged in anal sex with casual or regular partners (or both).

Knowledge of how many young heterosexuals are sexually active, the practices they engage in, and the number and type of partners cannot, alone provide an understanding of their risk of infection. Critical to an assessment of risk is knowledge of the extent to which sexual practices are 'safe' and, in particular, whether in penetrative sex condoms are used. Although there has been considerable increase in young people's acceptance of condoms during the past decade, studies of condom use show that most young people use condoms inconsistently or not at all (Dunne *et al.,* 1993; Gallois *et al.,* 1992; Rosenthal *et al.,* 1990; Rosenthal *et al.,* 1994; Turtle *et al.,* 1989; Weisberg, North & Buxton, 1992). The most common reason for girls' failure to use condoms is that they are on the contraceptive pill. Other common reasons are having trust in their partner and having a partner who is perceived to be 'clean'. There has, however, been an encouraging, albeit slow, increase in uptake of safe sex between 1990 and 1993 among the first-year university students surveyed annually by Crawford, Kippax, and Rodden (1994).

When young people do have multiple partners, they continue to make a distinction between casual and regular partners and there is evidence to suggest that sexual practices are modified accordingly. Overall, young people engage is less risky behaviours with casual partners than with regular partners. In particular, young women are more likely to use a condom if the sexual encounter is casual or does not occur 'in a relationship'. However, it is a concern that only a very short time span need elapse before a relationship is considered regular and that such an indiscriminate, flexible transition point may determine young women's use of condoms.

There are several recurring themes which arise from the research outlined above, and these provide the background information necessary for any understanding of young people's sexual behaviour. First, adolescence has frequently been portrayed as a period of sexual experimentation. While this is not true of all adolescents, there is certainly a pattern of sexual liberalism among some young people which involves high levels of casual sex, and multiple partners. Secondly, the number of young people who have used condoms each and every time they have had sex is extremely low.

KNOWLEDGE OF HIV/AIDS AND OTHER STDs

In early research, a key assumption was that unsafe sexual behaviour stemmed from a lack of knowledge about the transmission of HIV. If young people knew the consequences of unsafe sexual behaviour then they would not engage in these behaviours. By the mid 1990's most young people appear to be knowledgeable about HIV/AIDS but they do not appear to be applying their high levels of knowledge to their sexual practices. A number of studies, both in Australia and in other countries, have shown that higher levels of knowledge are unrelated to safe sex practices (Boldero, Moore, & Rosenthal, 1992; Kegeles, Adler & Irwin, 1988; Keller, *et al.,* 1988; Richard & van der Pligt, 1991; Weissman *et al.,* 1989).

The lack of a relationship between knowledge and behaviour has led some researchers to question the nature of the knowledge that young people have about HIV/AIDS. In interviews with young people, Slattery (1991) examined young teenagers' actual understanding of HIV/AIDS, as opposed to their ability to recite facts, and found a number of gaps. While most knew that sexual behaviour is associated with HIV transmission, and about two-thirds knew of the risks of contact with blood, few of these adolescents showed any understanding of the exact nature of the danger. For instance, many of these young people believed that contact with menstrual blood was more likely to give a person HIV than blood from a leg wound.

In another study, Rosenthal, Waters, and Glaun (1995) found that factual knowledge, assessed using a standard self-report questionnaire, was good, even among the youngest group studied (10 year-olds). However an interview revealed that many young people up to the age of 15 years who had high scores on the questionnaire demonstrated only a limited understanding of HIV/AIDS. Across all ages, understanding conformed to a developmental pattern that was consistent with these young people's cognitive level and with research on understanding of other illnesses (Glaun, 1991). The findings of these studies suggest that many young people do not have a high level of understanding of HIV/AIDS although they may have an adequate grasp of the relevant facts. This absence of true understanding may, in part, explain the reported lack of association between knowledge and behaviour change.

Little is known about young people's understanding of other STDs, despite the significant health threat that STDs pose. Dunne and his colleagues (Dunne *et al.*, 1993) found that high levels of knowledge about HIV transmission were not matched by knowledge of other STDs in high schoolers. While the most commonly named STD was herpes, less than half of the year 12 and less than one-third of the year 11 students named this disease. Chlamydia, currently an STD of considerable concern, was named by only 5% of year 12 boys and 19% of girls. Analogous findings were reported in a recent study which examined the knowledge of STDs in a large sample of Victorian high school students (Smith, Rosenthal, & Tesoriero, 1995) and in other studies (Wright, Gabb, & Ryan, 1991; Wyn, 1993).

In an older sample of 18 year-old tertiary students (Rosenthal & Moore, 1994) almost all had heard of HIV/AIDS, yet a large number had never heard of the other listed STDs (Chlamydia, gonorrhoea, herpes, and genital warts/HPV). Of those young people who had heard of these STDs, a large minority believed that they were either 'not very' or 'not at all' serious and did not have long-term consequences. Poor knowledge of STDs other than HIV was found in another study of Victorian university students (Minichiello, Paxton, Cowlings, *et al.*, 1994). It appears that the low levels of knowledge about STDs, identified among secondary school students, may persist into the late teen years.

SOURCES OF INFORMATION

Parents and Peers

We know that the perceived attitudes and values of significant others have an important shaping effect on an individual's intention to act in a particular manner and ultimately, on the performance of that action. Ajzen & Fishbein, 1977; Ajzen & Madden, 1986). Among adolescents, two such key influences are parents and peers. Moore and Rosenthal (1991a) reported that tertiary students perceived their parents as nonliberal in their sexual attitudes and relatively unlikely to discuss sex or safe sex with them, a finding confirmed by Stancombe (1994). Peers were regarded as more likely to discuss these matters than parents and as more liberal in their own sexual attitudes. Among younger adolescents, parents are infrequently used as sources of information about sexual matters, with both boys and girls being more confident that they could talk to people their own age about sex (Dunne *et al.*, 1993; Wright *et al.*, 1991).

In a study which examined parents' perceptions of the communication process, Rosenthal and Collis (in press) found that parents perceived themselves as being highly influential, relative to other information sources, on the knowledge and practices of their own 16 year-old adolescent. While almost all parents believed that they were open to discussions about sex, only two-thirds reported that they had actually discussed sexual matters with their teenage son or daughter. Ironically, these parents had an idealised view of their own teenager, and their relationship with him or her. Parents believe that their teenager is less sexually active than other teenagers, is more responsible about using condoms, more confident about sexual matters, more communicative with parents, and more influenced by parents than by other sources of sexual information. This idealistic vision needs to be interpreted in the context of an absence of widespread discussions about sex between parents and adolescents. In fact, parents' unrealistic views about their own adolescents and their contributions to young peoples' sex education, need to be challenged. The match or mismatch between young people's perceptions of their parents as communicators about sexual matters and that of the parents themselves needs to be negotiated.

Other sources

While parents and peers are important sources of information, they are not the only sources. Australian and international research has shown that the mass media are powerful sources of information about STDs for young people today (Abraham, Sheeran, Abrams, Spears & Marks, 1991; Harris, Harris & Davis, 1991; Stancombe, 1994; Wilders & MacCallum, 1990). While TV was the most common source of information for their high schoolers, Rosenthal and Smith (1995) found that the most trusted sources of information were those perceived as having 'legitimate' knowledge, namely health professionals, school sources, and information booklets. The finding that doctors are a trusted source of information who are rarely used points to the need to integrate health professionals into the education strategies used by young people. However, high trust in these sources is not matched by equally high preference for seeking them out. Wright *et al.,* (1991) report that a large majority of their teenagers would seek advice from the medical profession if they actually had symptoms or evidence of an infection with an STD, but very few would consult a health professional for preventive advice.

Paradoxically, the mass media, although the most common sources of information used by most students, lack credibility and are not well trusted. Clearly, high use of a particular information source should not be regarded as an indication that this source is effective. Rather, we must make accessible sources of information that young people prefer and trust and which are seen to have legitimate knowledge. It seems that there are some highly trusted sources (health professionals) who are not only not used, but also are unlikely to be accessed by choice. One potential avenue of providing readily available trusted sources is to extend the use of health professionals by commonly used media. For example, anecdotal evidence suggests that advice columns in magazines written by doctors have an impact on young girls, as do radio talk-back programs with doctors. Yet another strategy currently in place is to use medical students (a legitimate authority) who return to their schools to teach students about HIV/AIDS and other STDs.

ATTITUDES TO AIDS PREVENTION STRATEGIES

AIDS prevention campaigns have strongly promoted the need for consistent condom use among young people, with condoms being seen as the key to preventing the transmission of HIV among young people. There is evidence that the message 'safe sex equals condom use' has been well learned (Lenehan, Lynton, Bloom, & Blaxland, 1992; Stancombe, 1994) although some worrying alternative meanings were offered, such as having a 'clean partner', 'no fun, boring sex life', and monogamy. Few respondents mentioned non-penetrative sex as equating with safe sex and a substantial minority believed that safe/safer sex meant 'only having sex with your regular partner/not strangers'.

While there is evidence that some young people still have negative attitudes to condom use (Gallois *et al.*, 1992) encouraging reports from a number of Australian studies reveal positive attitudes (Crawford, Turtle, & Kippax, 1990; Moore & Rosenthal, 1991b). Reasons for negative attitudes to condoms vary. For some young people the issue is knowing how and where to buy the condoms, and feeling comfortable purchasing condoms. Hence there have been suggestions that condom use may be increased by making condoms more available through, for example, the installation of condom vending machines (Kashima, Gallois, & McCamish, 1992). For other young people the issue may not be the availability of condoms, but rather having negotiating skills required to convince sexual partners to agree to using them. Insisting that a partner use a condom, or to insist that this precaution is used oneself, may be seen to imply that the partner has an STD or be misconstrued as a lack of trust in the partner. Some young people dislike using condoms because they believe that sexual pleasure is reduced. Yet others feel that carrying condoms 'just in case', will reflect poorly on their reputation. In particular women may fear being labelled as 'easy' or 'a slut' if they carry condoms (Abbott, 1987).

Even if attitudes towards condoms are becoming more positive, this will not necessarily result in increased actual or intended use. Research that has examined the link between attitudes towards condoms and intentions to use them have found mixed results (Barling & Moore, 1991; Kashima, *et al.*, 1992; Boldero *et al.*, 1992). Intentions to use condoms in the future have been associated with both positive and negative attitudes, yet actual use has been found to depend on young people's negative attitudes to condoms, that is, the disadvantages of using condoms (Boldero *et al.*, 1992; Moore & Rosenthal, 1991b). In these studies, recognising the benefits of using condoms did not contribute significantly to actual condom use.

Of some concern is the evidence that, for most young people, condoms are still used as a contraceptive rather than as an STD precaution (Donald, Lucke, Dunne, O'Toole, & Raphael, in press; Robinson, 1993). Thus, when young women are using other contraceptive measures such as the pill or diaphragms, condoms are unlikely to be used as an additional disease prevention measure.

PERCEPTIONS OF RISK

Young people's behaviour is commonly regarded as being determined, at least in part, by the belief that they are invulnerable to the hazards that befall other individuals. This perceived sense of personal invulnerability to risk is of particular relevance to the study of young people's sexual risk-taking. It is clear that the sexual practices of many young people potentially place themselves and their partners at risk of STDs, including HIV. Whether, in fact, young people engage in these practices in spite of recognising their risky nature or whether they perceive, rightly or wrongly, their risk of infection to be low has been the focus of several studies.

Australian research confirms overseas findings that few heterosexual young people believe that HIV/AIDS is an issue relevant to their own lives. Adolescents of varying ages mostly perceive themselves to have a low risk of being infected with HIV/AIDS (Abbott, 1987; Crawford *et al.*, 1990; Gallois, Kashima, Hills & McCamish, 1990; Moore & Rosenthal, 1991c, 1992a; Wright, 1990).

The risk of being infected with other STDs is likewise perceived to be low (Lucke, Dunne, Donald, & Raphael, 1993). Moore and Rosenthal (1994) found that over half of the 18 year-old university students in their study considered themselves to be unlikely or extremely unlikely to contract an STD. However, these young people believed, realistically, that they were less likely to contract HIV than other STDs.

In some instances, young people's assessment of risk is appropriate in terms of their sexual practices. However, it seems that young people's perception of risk of HIV/AIDS and STDs is linked with other beliefs. These include having a stereotype of a person living with HIV/AIDS, feeling in control of whether or not they contracted HIV/AIDS, and whether they considered the prospect of having HIV/AIDS as highly undesirable (Moore & Rosenthal, 1991c). In part, what appears to be happening here is that young people have linked HIV/AIDS to risk-group rather than risk behaviours. A strong stereotype of a person with HIV/AIDS is likely to be maintained because few young people have ever known or met such a person. Given that, in Australia, social representations of people with HIV/AIDS focus on gay men, injecting drugs users, or sex workers, and in the absence of personal knowledge of someone with AIDS, it is likely that the stereotype that young people hold will be of someone unlike themselves. The stereotype serves a distancing function, especially since it enables individuals to focus on differences rather than possible similarities (eg. sexual practices) between themselves and whose who are infected.

The belief that becoming infected is something over which one has control serves to reduce perceptions of risk and suggests that issues of mastery and the ability to take responsibility for one's own sexuality are important in enabling young people to assess their risk realistically. Finally, a sense of invulnerability may be fostered by engaging in risky acts that do not have immediate negative consequences. This is especially problematic in the case of HIV infection. It is also true, given the epidemiology of HIV, that for most young people perceptions of low levels of risk are in fact accurate.

The research to date has mainly examined perceptions of HIV and STD risk independently of young people's more general risk environment. There is evidence that sexual risk-taking correlates with other risk-laden activities such as drinking, delinquent acts, and drug use (Jessor & Jessor, 1977), but the question of whether perceptions of risk associated with sexual activity from part of a more pervasive 'perception of risk environment' needs to be examined. In a recent study, Smith and Rosenthal (1995) demonstrated that adolescents' perceptions of risk are structured in readily interpretable ways. Unprotected sexual intercourse was rated as a high risk activity, along with driving a car while under the influence of drugs/alcohol, using inhalants, and taking amphetamines. Second-order factor suggested three overarching and independent components to young people's risk perception: the perceived danger of a particular activity, the risk payoff (which represents the tradeoff between pleasure obtained by engaging in the activity and peer approval/disapproval), and the focus of control.

By mapping the structure of young people's perceived risk environment, this study may provide a useful starting point for interventions to reduce adverse outcomes. If perceptions of risk in the sexual domain are embedded in a more generally structured risk environment, a broader-based approach to risk reduction may be an effective strategy. Certainly, recognition of risk is a positive step towards eventual change. The difficulty is to challenge the misguided beliefs that are associated with risky behaviours.

CONSTRUCTING SEXUALITY: BELIEFS AND COMPETENCIES

Recently there has been a shift away from documenting practices, knowledge, and attitudes to condoms among some researchers. The focus now is on the meanings that sexuality has for young men and women, and the ways in which these meanings are enacted in the context of relationships and sexual practice. An implicit corollary of this perspective is that rational decision-making models are unlikely to offer adequate explanations of sexual practices.

Thus, research has started with the premise that sexuality is a social construction. The many ways in which sexuality is conceptualised, defined, and expressed are determined by economic, political, and social forces rather than being the result of some 'natural' order of things. For example, recent studies which set young people's current sexual practices within the context of their understandings of sexuality (which in turn derive from social discourses around sexuality) have attempted to strip away the 'invisibility of heterosexuality'. In doing so, questions are asked about 'natural' sexual behaviour and the biological imperative which results in particular behaviours being regarded as appropriate and unchallenged for males and for females. By focussing on the context of sexual risk-taking, and setting sexual practices within broader notions of sexuality, researchers are able to augment correlational studies with insights drawn from young people's understandings of themselves as sexual beings, and the consequence of these understandings for sexual practices.

Some sexual myths

Young people's sense of invulnerability ('it can't happen to me') appears to be, for some, a powerful determinant of behaviour and has been discussed earlier. There are several other inappropriate beliefs or myths which have been identified. The first has been termed 'trusting to love' or the 'monogamy myth'. Many young people justify their non-use of condoms with the belief that their current relationship will be long-term and monogamous. Gallois, McCamish, and Kashima (1989) indicated that a majority of their sexually active heterosexuals kept themselves safe from infection by having sex only within what they believed to be an exclusive and monogamous relationship. Crawford *et al.*, (1990) also found that young heterosexuals were most likely to consider monogamy as a behaviour change that would protect them against HIV/AIDS infection. But relying on monogamy as a safe option is risky for at least two reasons. Many young people have a succession of permanent relationships of varying duration in which there is no sexual activity outside the relationship. This 'serial monogamy' entails much higher risks than long-term monogamy because each person may have a number of prior partners whose sexual history is not known. Second, as already noted, monogamy may not be adhered to by the partner, especially young men (Rosenthal *et al.*, 1990). The question that needs to be answered is whether their partners know that this is happening, or is likely to happen. If young people are making decisions about the type of sexual practices that are safe, based on an inaccurate understanding of their relationship (as they appear to be doing), then they are liable to place themselves at risk.

Another reason why some young people engage in unprotected sex with casual partners stems from a belief that you can tell if someone is infected by their appearance or reputation. (Chapman & Hodgson, 1988; Crawford *et al.*, 1990; Dunne *et al.*, 1993; Gold, Karmiloff-Smith, Skinner, & Morton, 1992) Young men are significantly more likely to employ this strategy of avoiding infection than women. There are several possible bases for the use of physical characteristics as a justification for unsafe sexual practices. First (and unlikely, given their generally high levels of knowledge about HIV/AIDS), these young people may not be aware of the long incubation period of HIV and thus that one cannot tell from appearances who is infected. Alternatively, they may be drawing incorrect inferences by generalising from frequently encountered diseases. Most diseases do, in fact, have short incubation periods so that one can tell by looking at a person whether they are infected. Or it is possible that these young people are simply drawing on the socially constructed equation of beauty and cleanliness with good health, assuming that only the ill-looking are ill.

Masculinity and femininity

Gender differences in young people's attitudes to sex are pervasive and influence their sexual practices. For example, there is a persistent belief in our society that men, unlike women, have an uncontrollable sex drive. Effectively, the male sex drive discourse (Holloway, 1984) serves to absolve young men of responsibility since 'they can't help themselves'.

Additional weight is given to the sexual imperative for young men in a study reported by Goggin (1989) in which young men were more likely than their female peers to report high levels of sexual arousal and desire for sexual exploration. Conversely, young women reported stronger belief in sexual commitment than did young men. As might be expected, high levels of arousal and exploration were associated with greater sexual risk-taking while high levels of commitment correlated with fewer sexual risks.

It appears, too, that young girls have different emotional responses to sexual intercourse than boys, following both their first and subsequent sexual experiences (Donald, Lucke, Dunne & Raphael, in press; McCabe & Collins, 1990), with girls more likely than boys to report negative emotions such as feeling bad or 'used', the more so if they were drunk or high at the time, or had sex with someone who was not a steady partner. Added weight to the conclusion that sex, for some girls, is not pleasurable, comes in a recent qualitative study (Stewart, 1994). While these girls describe sex as "boring", they give a positive account of erotic foreplay, suggesting that the 'paradigmatic shift' from penetrative to non-penetrative sex (Wilton & Aggleton, 1991) may not be an unrealistic goal, at least for girls.

When young people are asked about their reasons for having or not having sex, girls were more likely than boys to say that they had not met the right person or were not ready. Boys were more likely to say that they hadn't had the opportunity. Love, caring, and affection were girls' primary motivation for engaging in sex. This was a less common reason for boys, a substantial number of whom said that they engaged in sex for physical pleasure (Rosenthal *et al.,* 1994). These responses may well reflect norms about gender. Young girls may be reasoning that they need to be in 'love' as a justification for engaging in sex; young boys may be willing to admit to a motive that fits with a norm of male sex as urgent and exploratory.

Young women's focus on love and relationships rather than sex is a finding common to other studies (eg., Roberts, Kippax, Waldby, & Crawford, in press; Stancombe, 1994). Roberts *et al.,* in a paper exploring the faking of orgasm by young women and the reasons underlying this practice, comment on their female participants' focus on love and relationships rather than the physical aspects of sex. In contrast, for young men sexual activity is conceptualised in terms of 'work' and 'technique'. Having a woman orgasm, then, is evidence for successful technique or work satisfactorily completed. Women must demonstrate the value of this 'work', these writers argue, by having an orgasm, imagined or real.

The traditional interpretation of masculinity offers men greater power than women in gender relationships. In the sexual domain this position is manifested by a masculine preference for controlling the initiative (Kippax, Crawford, & Waldby, 1994; Waldby, Kippax, and Crawford (1993). As Kippax *et al.,* point out, while this stance does not necessarily preclude safe sex, it does make it difficult for young women to have their say and be heard. Thus, masculinity norms operate to reinforce the power differential around sexuality, including the nature of relationships. Control in the sexual sphere is exercised by men and young women learn to operate within this framework. In drawing this conclusion, Waldby and her colleagues add a cautionary note. While many (most)? young men act out this controlling role in sexual relationships, there is a substantial minority who express fears and concerns about their sexuality and about their sexual competence. This point is exemplified by some of the young men in Buzwell's research (see below).

Confidence and communication

Asked questions relating to their confidence in communicating their wishes in sexual situations, the majority of Dunne *et al.*'s high schoolers claimed that they could negotiate the most responsible outcome. Given the likelihood that many of those claiming to be confident had never experienced the situation in question (eg. persuading an unwilling partner to use a condom), these figures may overestimate the reality. Rosenthal, Moore, and Flynn (1991) found that confidence in 18 years-olds' ability to deal with sexual matters and sexual self-esteem varied by gender and according to the aspect of sexuality being addressed. Most young people were confident that they could purchase condoms and discuss their use, and delay sex until precautions were available, although a substantial minority lack confidence in their ability to purchase condoms and report that they do not know how to use a condom.

Those who were more confident in dealing with sexual matters were engaging in safer sexual practices with both regular and casual partners for both sexes. The authors suggest that the gender differences in absolute levels of confidence and self-worth add weight to the conclusion that young men and women bring different competencies to the sexual encounter. However, they note that confidence in their ability to deal with sexual precautions was not associated with young people's sexual practices, cautioning that the spontaneous nature of much sexual activity may militate against effective preparation for safe sex.

Communication with a partner about sex has two important functions. It allows for discussion of a partner's sexual history and for negotiations about safe sex. Certainly, communication with a partner about the desire to have safe sex (ie. use a condom) has been implicated as a critical factor in achieving this goal (eg. Boldero *et al.,* 1992; Kashima *et al.,* 1992). In these studies, having communicated about using a condom was an important determinant of whether or not a condom was actually used. While the majority of students in the national study of high schoolers (Dunne *et al.,* 1993) reported that they talked to their partner about condom use last time they had sex, many did not, casting some doubt on the professed confidence of these young people in their ability to discuss condom use (and other matters of relevance) with their partners.

Constructing a sexual identity

A recent approach to conceptualising sexual practices has been to link these with the ways in which young people construct a sense of their sexual identity. These studies examine the ways in which beliefs about themselves as sexual beings come together to form a sexual 'style' or 'ideology' which influences their behaviour in the sexual arena. Moore and Rosenthal (1992) identified a number of themes which encapsulated 16 year-olds' sexual worlds. These included a permissive attitude to sexuality, wherein premarital sex and one-night-stands were regarded as acceptable, a recognition that double standards still exist, where what is appropriate and acceptable sexual behaviour for boys (eg. casual sex) is not for girls, a view of sex equating with romance (mostly held by girls), and, in contrast, a sexually aggressive, exploitative theme expressed by some boys. While some young people's constructions of sexuality were consistent throughout their interviews, others demonstrated inconsistencies and contradictions as they tried to establish a position for themselves on this issue.

Buzwell (Buzwell & Rosenthal, 1996) has delineated five distinct sexual styles among a homogeneous group of high schoolers. These styles reflect a constellation of beliefs and attitudes about sexuality, including those who are sexually unassured, idealistic, competent, adventurous, or driven. There are gender differences in styles, with more young girls than boys in the idealistic group and approximately equal numbers in the competent group. As might be expected, the adventurous and driven groups are almost entirely composed of young boys. Buzwell found membership of a style was associated with sexual behaviours. For example, the first two groups consisted mostly of virgins, while the last two were associated with higher levels of sexual risk-taking.

This holistic approach to understanding young people's sexual attitudes and beliefs has considerable potential in aiding the development of educational programs. Broad education programs have an important role to play, but there should be also the opportunity for interventions which are tailored for particular subgroups of young people. There is a need to understand the way in which young people are conceptualising their sexual experiences, in order to target them effectively. For example, different education programs are likely to be effective for 'invulnerable' adolescents and for the aware risk-takers. Those young women who 'trust to love' will need to receive different messages from those who believe that attractiveness equals safety.

CONCLUSION

The advent of HIV/AIDS as a serious threat to young people and the community at large has resulted in considerable energy being directed towards preventing a single STD. While other STDs do not have such uniformly adverse outcomes as HIV, their greater incidence, prevalence and consequent morbidity among adolescents and young adults requires that more resources be developed to address the educational needs of young people in this respect. An increase in knowledge about the more prevalent STDs amongst young people is likely to increase their perception of risk as a result of knowing an infected person. This may then result in safer behaviour which inadvertently decreases risk of HIV.

Substantial resources have been allocated to educating young people to adopt safe sexual practices, including national media campaigns, school-based education programs, and other community initiatives. Cohort studies have provided evidence of only modest change, suggesting that, while there has been a gradual shift in the culture around safe sex, there is still a long way to go. Mapping young people's sexuality in all its complexity and shades of meaning should result in programs which will enable young people to negotiate sex safely and maintain their sexual well-being.

REFERENCES

Abbott, S. (1987) Talking about AIDS: A report on the issues of AIDS with young women. *AIDS Action Council*, Canberra.

Abraham, C., Sheeran, P., Abrams, D., Spears, R., & Marks, D. (1991) Young people learning about AIDS: A study of beliefs and information sources. *Health Education Research*, **6**, 19-29.

Ajzen, I. & Fishbein, M. (1977) Attitude-behaviour relations: A theoretical analysis and review of empirical research. *Psychological Bulletin*, **84**, 888-919.

Ajzen, I & Madden, T.J. (1986) Prediction of goal-directed behaviour: Attitudes, intentions and perceived behavioural control. *Journal of Experimental and Social Psychology*, **22**, 453-474.

Barling, N.R., & Moore, S.M. (1991) Adolescents' attitudes towards AIDS precautions and intention to use condoms. *Psychological Reports*, **67**, 883-890.

Boldero, J.M., Moore, S.M., & Rosenthal, D.A. (1992) Intention, context, and safe sex: Australian adolescents' response to AIDS. *Journal of Applied Social Psychology*, **22**, 1357-1397.

Brooks-Gunn, J. & Furstenberg, F.F. Jr. (1989) Adolescent sexual behaviour. *American Psychologist*, **44**, 249-257.

Buzwell, S. & Rosenthal, D.A. (1996) Constructing a sexual self: Adolescents' sexual self perceptions and sexual risk taking. *Journal of Research on Adolescence*, **6**(4), 489-513.

Chapman, S. & Hodgson, J. (1988) Showers in raincoats: Attitudinal barriers to condom use in high risk heterosexuals. *Community Health Studies*, **12**, 97-105.

Crawford, J., Turtle, A.M., & Kippax, S. (1990) Student favoured strategies for AIDS prevention strategies. *Australian Journal of Psychology*, **42**, 123-138.

Crawford, J., Kippax, S., & Rodden, P. (1994) Knowledge and safe practice among heterosexual tertiary students as an outcome of sociocultural change. *Paper presented at the Xth International AIDS Conference Yokohama, Japan, August.*

Donald, M., Lucke, J., Dunne, M., & Raphael, B. (in press) Gender differences associated with young peoples' emotional reactions to intercourse. *Journal of Youth and Adolescence.*

Donald, M. Lucke, J., Dunne, M., O'Toole, B., & Raphael, B. (in press) Determinants of condom use by Australian secondary students. *Journal of Adolescent Health.*

Donovan, B. (1992). After a decade of AIDS are the other STDs still relevant? *Today's Life Science*, December.

Dunne, M., Donald, M., Lucke, J., & Raphael, B. (in press) The sexual behaviour of young people in rural Australia. In K. Malko (Ed.), *Proceedings of the Second National Rural Health Conference.* Canberra: Department of Health, Housing and Community Services.

Dunne, M., Donald, M., Lucke, J. *et al.*, (1994) Age-related increase in sexual behaviours and decrease in regular condom use among adolescents in Australia. *International Journal of STDs and AIDS*, **5**, 41-47.

Gallois, C., McCamish, M., & Kashima, Y. (1989) *Safe and unsafe sexual practices by heterosexuals and homosexual men: Predicting intentions and behaviour*, University of Queensland Press.

Gallois, C., Kashima, Y., Hills, R., & McCamish, M. (1990) Preferred strategies for safe sex: Relation to past and actual behaviour among sexually active men and women. *Paper presented at the Sixth International Conference on AIDS*, San Francisco, June.

Gallois, C., Kashima, Y., Terry, D., McCarnish, M., Timmins, P., & Chauvin, A. (1992) Safe and unsafe sexual intentions and behaviour: The effects of norms and attitudes. *Journal of Applied Social Psychology*, **22**, 1521-1545.

Garland, S.M., Gertig, M., & Mclnnes, J.A. (1993) Genital Chlamydia trachomatis infection in Australia. *The Medical Journal of Australia*, **159**, 90-96.

Glaun, D. (1991). *Development of CF and the healthy children's concepts of illness and the body.* Unpublished PhD thesis, University of Melbourne, Melbourne, Australia.

Gold, R.S. Karmiloff-Smith, A., Skinner, M.J., & Morton, J. (1992) Situational factors and thought processes associated with unprotected intercourse in heterosexual students. *AIDS Care*, **4**, 305-323.

Goggin, M. (1989) *Intimacy, sexuality, and the sexual behaviour among young Australian adults.* Unpublished B.A. (Hons.) thesis, Department of Psychology, University of Melbourne, Australia.

Goldman, R.J., & Goldman, J.D.G. (1988) *Show me yours: Understanding children's sexuality.* Ringwood: Penguin.

Harris, M.B. Harris, R.J., & Davis, S.M. (1991) Ethnic and gender differences in Southwestern students' sources of information about health. *Health Education Research*, **6**, 31-42.

Hart, G. (1993) The epidemiology of genital chlamydial infection in South Australia. *International Journal of STD and AIDS*, **4**, 204-210.

Hein, K. (1989) AIDS in adolescence: A rationale for concern. *New York State Journal of Medicine*, **87**, 290-295.

Hofferth, S.L. & Hayes, C.D. (1987) *Risking the future: Adolescent sexuality, pregnancy and childbearing 1*, Washington DC: National Academy of Science.

Holloway, W. (1984) Women's power in heterosexual sex. *Women's Studies International Forum*, 7, 66-68.

Jessor, S.L., & Jessor, R. (1977) *Problem behaviour and psychological development: A longitudinal study of youth.* New York: Academic Press.

Kashima, Y., Gallois, C., & McCamish, M. (1992) Predicting the use of condoms: Past behaviour, norms and the sexual partner. In T. Edgar, M.A. Fitzpatrick, & V.S. Freimuth (Eds.), *AIDS: A communication perspective* (pp. 21-46). Hillsdale, NJ: Lawrence Erlbaum.

Kegeles, S., Adler, N., & Irwin, C. (1988) Sexually active adolescents and condoms: Knowledge, attitudes and changes over one year. *American Journal of Public Health*, **78**, 260-261.

Keller, S.E. Schleifer, S.J. Bartlett, J.A. & Johnson, R.L. (1988) The sexual behaviour of adolescents and risk of AIDS. *Journal of the American Medical Association*, **260**, 5386.

Kippax, S., Crawford, J., & Waldby, C. (1994) Heterosexuality, masculinity and HIV: Barriers to safe heterosexual practice. *AIDS Special Supplement.*

Kovacs, G.T., Westcott, M., Rusden, J. *et al.*, (1987) The prevalence of Chlamydia trachomatis in a young sexually active population. *The Medical Journal of Australia.* **147**, 550-552.

Lenehan, Lynton, Bloom & Blaxland, (1992) *Exploring what youth understands 'safe sex' and 'safer sex' to mean.* Lenehan, Lynton, Bloom & Blaxland, Sydney.

Loxley, W. & Ovenden (1992) "I wouldn't share": Teenage injecting drug users in Perth and HIV/AIDS prevention. *Paper presented at the 3rd International Conference on the Reduction of Drug Related Harm.*

Lucke, J., Dunne, M., Donald, M., & Raphael, B. (1993) Knowledge of STDs and perceived risk of infection: A study of Australian youth, *Venereology*, **6**, 57-63.

McCabe, M. & Collins, J. (1990) *Dating, relating and sex.* Sydney: Horowitz Grahame.

Minichiello, V., Paxton, S. Cowlings, V. *et al.*, (1994) Young people's knowledge of STDs: Labels, transmission and symptoms. *Paper presented at the Australasian Sexual Health Conference*, Queensland, April.

Moore, S.M. & Rosenthal, D.A. (1991a) Adolescents' perceptions of friends' and parents' attitude to sex and sexual risk-taking. *Journal of Community and Applied Psychology.* **1**, 189-200.

Moore, S.M. & Rosenthal, D.A. (1991c) Adolescent invulnerability and perception of AIDS risk. *Journal of Adolescent Research*, **6**, 164-180.

Moore, S.M. & Rosenthal, D.A. (1992) The social context of adolescent sexuality: Safe sex implications. *Journal of Adolescence*, **15**, 1-21.

Moore, S.M. & Rosenthal, D.A. (1994) Young people assess their risk of sexually transmissible diseases. *Psychology and Health*, **10**, 17-31.

Richard, R & van der Pligt, J. (1991) Factors affecting condom use among adolescents. *Journal of Community and Applied Social Psychology*, **1**, 105-116.

Robinson, J. (Ed). (1993) *"Becoming aware...": Women and HIV/AIDS.* Deakin, ACT: Family Planning Australia.

Roberts, C., Kippax, S., Spongberg, M., & Crawford, J. (in press) 'Going down': Oral sex, imaginary bodies and HIV. *AIDS and Culture.*

Roberts, C., Kippax, S. Waldby, C., & Crawford, J. (in press) Faking it: The story of "OHHI". *Womens Studies International Forum.*

Rollins, B. (1989) *Sexual attitudes and behaviours: A review of the literature.* Melbourne: Australian Institute of Family Studies.

Rosenthal, D.A. & Collis, F. (in press) Parents' beliefs about adolescent sexuality and HIV/AIDS. *Journal of HIV Education and Prevention in Children and Adolescents.*

Rosenthal, D.A., Moore, S.M. & Brumen, I. (1990) Ethnic group differences in adolescents' responses to AIDS. *Australian Journal of Social Issues.* **25**, 220-239.

Rosenthal, D.A. Moore, S.M. & Buzwell, S. (1994) Homeless youths: Sexual and drug related behaviour, sexual beliefs and HIV/AIDS risk. *AIDS Care*, **6**, 83-94.

Rosenthal, D.A., Moore, S.M., & Flynn, I. (1991) Adolescent self-efficacy, self-esteem and sexual risk taking. *Journal of Community and Applied Social Psychology.* **1**, 77-88.

Rosenthal, D.A., & Moore, S.M. (1994) Stigma and ignorance: Young people's beliefs about STDs. *Venereology*, 7, 62-68.

Rosenthal, D.A. Waters, L., & Glaun, D. (1995) What do pre-adolescents understand about HIV/AIDS? *Psychology and Health*, **10**, 507-522

Rosenthal, D.A. & Smith, A.M. (1995) Adolescents and sexually transmissible diseases: Information sources, preferences and trust. *Health Promotion Journal of Australia*, **5**, 38-44.

Short, R.V. (1993) The AIDS Epidemic: What are the Priorities? *Paper presented at the VIIIth World Congress on Human Reproduction*, Bali, Indonesia, April.

Slattery, M. (1991) Adolescents knowledge and understanding of AIDS related concepts. *Paper presented at the International Conference on Health Education*, Helsinki.

Smith, A.M.A. & Rosenthal, D.A. (1995) Adolescents' perceptions of their risk environment. *Journal of Adolescence*, **18**, 229-245

Smith, A.M.A., Rosenthal, D.A., & Tesoriero, A. (1995) Adolescents and sexually transmissible diseases: Patterns of knowledge in Victorian high schools. *Venereology*, **8**, 83-88.

Stancombe (1994) *Qualitative Research Findings on Young Heterosexuals: The 1994 Communication Environment in the Context of Sexually Transmitted Diseases including HIV/AIDS.* Prepared for Research and Marketing Group Public Affairs Branch.

Stevenson, E. (Ed.). (1993) Surveillance of Sexually Transmissible Diseases in Victoria 1992. *Victoria: AIDS/STD Unit,* Department of Health and Community Services Victoria.

Stevenson, F., Gertig, D., Crofts, N., Sherrard, J., Forsyth, J., & Breschkin, A. (1992) Three potential spectres of youth: Chlamydia, Gonorrhoea and HIV and Victorian youth, January 1991 to June 1992. *Paper presented at the Australian Scientific congress on Sexually Transmissible Diseases,* Sydney, November.

Stewart, F. (1994) 'they think it comes in a package deal...' Young rural and urban women's negotiation of their sexual lives. *Paper presented at the HIV, AIDS and Society Conference,* Sydney, July.

Turtle, A.M., Ford, B., Habgood, R. *et al.,* (1989) AIDS related beliefs and behaviours of Australian university students. *Medical Journal of Australia.* **150**, 371-376.

Waldby, C., Kippax, S., & Crawford, J. (1993) Research note: Heterosexual men and 'safe sex' practice. *Sociology of Health and Illness.* **15**, 246-256.

Wasserheit, J.N. (1992) Interrelationships between human immunodeficiency virus infection and other sexually transmitted diseases. *Sexually Transmitted Diseases.* **19**, 61-77.

Weisberg, E., North, P., & Buxton, M. (1992) Sexual activity and condom use in high school students. *Medical Journal of Australia,* **156**, 612-613.

Weissman, C., Nathanson, C., Ensminger, M., Robinson, J., & Plitcha, S. (1989) AIDS knowledge, perceived risk, and prevention among adolescent clients attending a family planning clinic. *Family Planning Perspectives.* **21**, 213-217.

Wright, B. (1990) *Student perceptions of AIDS: Seriousness and personal risk assessments.* University of Queensland.

Wright, S.M. Gabb. R.G. & Ryan, M.M. (1991) Reproductive health: Knowledge, attitudes and needs of adolescents. *Medical Journal of Australia,* **155**, 325-328.

Wilders, S. & MacCallum, M. (1990) *Research Report: Women and AIDS.* Report prepared by Power Research for the Department of Community Services and Health, Canberra.

Wilton, T. & Aggleton, P. (1991) Condoms, coercion and control: Heterosexuality and the limits to HIV/AIDS education. In P. Aggleton., G. Hart., & P. Davies (Eds.). *AIDS: Responses, Interventions and care.* London: Falmer Press.

Wyn, J. (1993) Young women's health: The challenge of sexually transmitted diseases. *Working Paper No. 8, Youth Research Centre,* Institute of Education, University of Melbourne, Australia.

8

Adolescents and HIV Risk Due to Drug Injection or Sex with Drug Injectors in the United States

SAMUEL R. FRIEDMAN, ALAN NEAGUS, BENNY JOSE, RICHARD CURTIS, GENE A. McGRADY, MILDRED VERA, RICHARD LOVELY, JONATHAN ZENILMAN, VALERIE JOHNSON, HELENE R. WHITE, DENISE PAONE & DON C. DES JARLAIS

INTRODUCTION

Although many young adults are at behavioural risk of becoming infected with human immunodeficiency virus (HIV) (Catania *et al.,* 1992), the extent of HIV infection among heterosexual adolescents and young adults in the United States still appears to be limited in comparison to the extent of pregnancy and other sexually transmitted diseases (STDs) among them. We do not fully understand the processes that shape the HIV epidemic among youth. Their high prevalence of STDs and pregnancies suggests the possibility that HIV seroprevalence among them could increase greatly, but the relatively low HIV prevalence among youth in New York – a city in which HIV has been widespread among gay and bisexual men, and among drug injectors, for fifteen years or more – suggests the possibility that social conditions or other factors in economically developed countries, such as the United States, might restrain heterosexual HIV transmission.

Thus, we need a better understanding of how HIV and STDs spread among youth. In part, the answer to this is evident – HIV and other infections spread through unprotected sex with an infected person and/or through injecting drugs with infected syringes. However, saying this leads to several important additional questions: First, what patterns of social relationships and other factors predispose some youth to engage in high risk behaviour? Second, why do some youth engage in risk behaviour with infected persons and other not? Third, how do the overall patterns of risk behaviours and risk relationships produce observed rates of infection? And fourth, what processes might lead to, or prevent, greatly increased HIV infection rates among youth?

This chapter cannot answer these questions. What it does do is to review some of the evidence about rates of infection, among youth, by HIV and by other diseases that can be transmitted sexually or through drug injection. (In doing this, we focus to some extent upon New York City, precisely because HIV has been very widespread among gay/bisexual men and among drug injectors there, which makes it easier to detect potential spread of HIV from these groups to heterosexual non-drug-injecting youth.) Then, the chapter focuses on the risk of becoming a drug injector and actual and potential sexual relationships with drug injectors. We present a theoretical model of some ways in which youth become drug injectors, and discuss some of the research which supports this model. We then turn to a brief discussion of preliminary results from research projects that are studying the social and risk networks of youth in three cities (New York, Atlanta, and San Juan), and use this research to help interpret the infection rates presented earlier in the chapter. Finally, while recognizing that current knowledge is extremely limited, we suggest some possible ways in which the further spread of HIV among youth might be slowed.

RATES OF INFECTION WITH HIV AND OTHER AGENTS THAT CAN BE TRANSMITTED VIA DRUG INJECTION OR SEX

AIDS surveillance data suggest that a large number of adolescents and young adults in the United States have been infected with HIV. By June, 1994, cumulative AIDS cases added up to 1,768 among 13-19 years olds; 15,204 among 20-24 years olds; and 60,041 among 25-29 year olds (Centers for Disease Control, 1994). Most of the AIDS cases among 13-19 year-old men are ascribed either to male/male sex (33%) or to having been infused with infected blood products (44%) during treatment for hemophilia/blood coagulation disorder prior to the introduction of effective methods for screening blood products and killing HIV in blood donations.

Table 1
The Proportions (and Numbers) of Adolescent and Young Adult AIDS cases in the United States of America that have been among persons who have injected drugs but who have not engaged in male/male sex*.

Age	Male	Female
13-19	7% (79)	19% (105)
20-24	13% (1,505)	34% (1,121)

* Cases reported to the Centers for Disease Control and Prevention through June 1994. Among males, an additional 4% of cases among 13-19 year-olds and 11% of cases among 20-24 year-olds are among persons who have both injected drugs and engaged in male/male sex.

Among 20-24 year old men, male/male sex accounts for 64% of AIDS cases (and hemophilia/coagulation-related transmission for only 4%). The proportion of AIDS cases in these age categories among persons who have injected drugs is presented in Table 1. Approximately half of the cases among young women, but only one-fortieth of those among young men, are ascribed to heterosexual transmission; and approximately half of the heterosexual transmission cases report that they have had sex with a drug injector. (Since the source of risk for AIDS cases depends primarily on self-report, there may be a tendency to under-report certain stigmnatized behaviours, such as drug injecting and homosexual activity, and to overestimate the proportion of cases due to heterosexual transmission.) Given the latency period between infection and diagnosis (which can be formalized through back-calculation {Gayle & D'Angelo, 1991}), these date indicate that many youth are becoming infected during their teenage years or shortly thereafter.

A number of studies have been conducted to determine HIV infection rates among youth. Back-calculation methods indicate that about 17,000 United States teenagers (ages 13-19) were infected with HIV from 1981 through 1987 (Gayle & D'Angelo, 1991). Bowler *et al.* (1992) review data from a wide variety of adolescent seroprevalence surveys at STD clinics, women's health centers, Job Corps entrants, military testing units, hospitals, a New York City homeless shelter, and a family planning clinic. Here, we will emphasize the data for New York because, as Bowler *et al.* (1992) argue, HIV risk is greatest for teens (and young adults) "in communities where HIV infection is common." These data find seroprevalence rates up to 5.3% among homeless and runaway youth (aged 15-22) in the New York City homeless shelter study. Among non-IDU women getting first trimester abortions in a New York medical center (Schoenbaum *et al.*, 1989), rates of 1.8% were found for subjects aged 15-19 and 2.5% for those aged 20-24. Among Kings County (Brooklyn) youth less than 20 years of age who applied for entry into the US military, only 0.2% were seropositive (Burke *et al.*, 1990). Unfortunately, most of these studies collect little information about behaviours and almost no information about youth's social and risk networks. Thus, far more remains to be learned about behavioural and associational patterns that put adolescents and young adults at risk for HIV.

Widespread sexual activity without condoms means that many adolescents and young adults who have not yet become infected are at sexual risk for HIV, and that successive cohorts will become so as they reach the age at which they become sexually active. The extent of this risk is indicated by the high rate of pregnancy among 15-17 year old women (over 70/1,000 in 1985 {DHHS 1991}). Early age of first sexual intercourse is associated with increasing numbers of sex partners and with higher risk for STDs (Zelnick, Kantner & Ford, 1981). The proportion of adolescent women who have engaged in sexual intercourse by any given age has increased rapidly since 1970, and by 1988 was about 26% by age 15, 32% by 16, 51% by 17, 69% by 18, and 75% by 19 (Centers for Disease Control, 1991).

STD rates provide additional data on the extent of risk. Nationally, 15-19 year olds have the highest rates of chlamydial cervicitis, gonorrhea, and for females, pelvic inflammatory disease hospitalizations (Aral *et al.*, 1988; Bell & Hein, 1984;

Kipke *et al.,* 1990). Reported cases of syphilis have been rising in the United States – particularly among African Americans. Rates of reported cases per 100,000 for 1991 were, among 15-19 year olds, 26 for syphilis, 7.5 for hepatitis B, and 894 for gonorrhea; and for 20-24 year olds, 50 for syphilis, 14 for hepatitis B, and 893 for gonorrhea (Centers for Disease Control, 1992). These data indicate that many youth engage in high-risk behaviour that could transmit HIV; they also indicate a widespread potential vulnerability to STD-facilitated HIV transmission (Hook *et al.,* 1992a, 1992b, Jones & Wasserheit, 1991; Padian, Shibosky & Hitchcock, 1991).

Preliminary data is available from a household survey of 18-21 year old youth that we are conducting in the Bushwick section of Brooklyn NY. This is a neighbourhood of working class and unemployed people, many of them Latino or African/American and thus subjected to the racial subordination that characterizes American society (Geschwender, 1978). There are thousands of drug injectors in the neighbourhood, of whom approximately 40% are HIV-infected and 70% have been infected with hepatitis B (Friedman *et al.,* in press), which would indicate that there is a serious risk of widespread sexual diffusion of infections from drug injectors to other people – including youth – in the neighbourhood. Our preliminary data indicate that the following proportions of youth have been infected with various infectious agents:

Table 2
Infection Rates among Youth in Bushwick

Infection	Number of youth tested	Number infected	Percent infected	95% Confidence Interval
HIV	58	0	0%	0 - 5.1%
Hepatitis C	65	0	0%	0 - 4.5%
Human T-Cell Lymphotropic Virus, Type I	63	0	0%	0 - 4.6%
Human T-Cell Lymphotropic Virus, Type II	58	0	0%	0 - 5.1%
Hepatitis B	58	2	3.4%	0 - 8.1%
Chlamydia	35	7	20%	7-33%
Herpes Simplex, type 2	50	17	34%	21-47%

Researchers in a hospital in another part of Brooklyn studied a predominantly (90%) Black sample of sexually active women aged 18-50 who had never injected drugs. Forty-two percent of the women aged 18 and 19, and 49% of those 20-24, were positive for herpes simplex virus type 2 (DeHovitz *et al.,* 1992). Age, number of sex partners in the past year, and cocaine use were significant risk factors for HSV-2, and condom use the last time the subject had sex was a significant protective factor.

HOW HETEROSEXUAL YOUTH COME TO BE AT RISK FOR HIV THROUGH DRUG INJECTION OR THROUGH SEXUAL NETWORKS INCLUDING DRUG INJECTORS

There has been considerable research that helps us to understand how some youth come to be at risk for HIV, although much additional research is needed. This research is discussed below. Figure 1 presents a model of the process as we understand it. It will be discussed "backwards," starting from the outcome (infection) and working backwards.

Infection occurs as the result of a high-risk behaviour being enacted with a partner who is infected. Thus, infection rates are determined both by the frequency of high-risk behaviours and by the probability that one or more partners is infected – and, in addition, by their interaction terms (Friedman *et al.*, 1993; Neaigus *et al.*, 1994, 1995).

Potential determinants of (a) risk behaviours and (b) involvement in high risk social networks include sociodemographic factors and personal and interpersonal variables such as childhood conduct disorder, family relationships, or having been sexually abused. Of central importance is the problematic use of alcohol and other drugs, which may be key determinants of sexual and drug risk behaviours (Stinson *et al.*, 1992) and also may play a major role in shaping youths' social networks. Furthermore, much of the impact of sociodemographic and other antecedent variables is likely to be mediated through subjects' alcohol and other drug use.

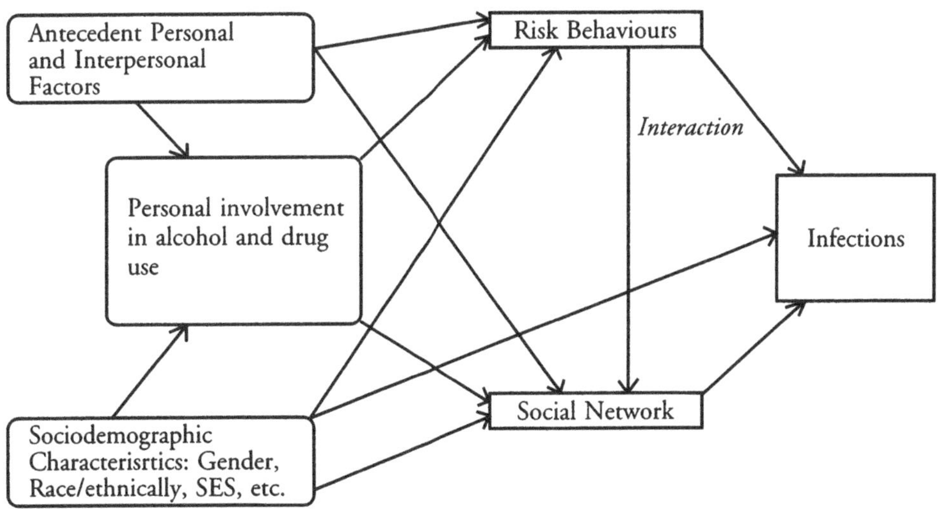

Fig. 1

Risk Behaviours, Social Networks, and Infection

The immediate causes of infection with HIV or other pathogens discussed in this chapter are likely to involve drug injection or sexual behaviours. Drug injection using shared equipment or drug mixtures can transmit HIV, HTLV-I, HTLV-II, HBV, and HCV. Unprotected sex can transmit HIV, HBV, HSV-2, chlamydia, gonorrhea, and probably HTLV-I (Gorbach *et al.,* 1993). The probability of infection due to high-risk behaviours, however, is affected by the probability that a drug-injection partner or sex partner is infected. For example, new injectors are more likely to become infected with HIV if they engage in high risk behaviours and if their drug injecting networks contain IDUs who are likely to be infected (Friedman *et al.,* 1993; Neaigus *et al.,* 1994). Other aspects of social networks can also affect the probability of infection with HIV or other sexually-transmitted diseases (Friedman *et al.,* in press(a); Klovdahl *et al.,* 1994; Neaigus *et al.,* 1995; Potterat, 1992).

Links from "Gateway" Substance Use to Risk Behaviours and Social Networks

As is discussed below, there appears to be a pattern in the use of mood-altering substances. Few persons come to use or to inject drugs such as heroin or cocaine without using marijuana or other "softer" drugs first; and few persons use these softer drugs without using alcohol and/or tobacco first (Kandel *et al.,* 1992). Of course, most people who use alcohol and other 'soft' drugs do not go on to 'hard' drug use. Rather, it is the intensity with which these drugs are used, and the precocity of their use, i.e., the early age at which they are used, which makes them more likely to function as gateways to using or injecting heroin or cocaine. Thus, it is worthwhile considering some of the evidence that the use of alcohol and "softer" drugs is related to infections, to risk behaviours and risk networks. *Alcohol Use and Infections:* Alcohol use has been linked to sexually – and parenterally – transmitted infection. Shafer *et al.* (1993) found adolescent male detainees who reported current daily use to be more likely to have had an STD (odds ratio = 3.53) than current non-users. Ericksen & Trocki (1992) found that problem drinking was associated in multivariate analysis with self-reported STDs among both adult men and women. *Alcohol Use and Sexual Risk Behaviours:* The link between alcohol use and sex can be approached in two ways. One is developmentally (see the discussion below of Predictors of Problem Drinking and Other Problem Behavior.) The other is in terms of whether alcohol use makes it more likely that one will engage in a particular episode of unprotected sexual behaviour. On this event-specific level, several mechanisms have been proposed: (1) Alcohol may lower inhibitions, leading to unplanned or unprotected sex (Denzin, 1987): (2) Sexual intentions may cause alcohol use, either because people who want to have sex (particularly with a new partner) may engage in alcohol use as a way to relieve their anxiety (Klassen & Wilsnack, 1986) or as a way to provide themselves with an excuse to take sexual risks (Cooper, 1992); (3) Some predisposing personality trait or conduct problem may lead to both alcohol use and high-risk sexual behaviour.

Although some studies find that drinking is not related to high-risk sex (Bolton *et al.,* 1992; Leigh, 1990; Martin & Hasin, 1990; Temple & Leigh, 1992), most published reports suggest that there is at least a statistical association between drinking and sex. Keller *et al.* (1991) assessed sexual risk behaviours among healthy inner city adolescents recruited in clinics and high school. They found that even moderate levels of alcohol or marijuana use predicted high risk sexual behaviours. Strunin & Hingson (1992) found that Massachusetts adolescents were more likely to have sex if they or their partner had been drinking and less likely to use condoms after drinking. Gillmore *et al.* (1992) found that alcohol use was associated with high risk sexual behaviour among female adolescents. O'Leary *et al.* (1992) found that safer sex was less likely among college students who combine sex with alcohol or drug use, as did Clapper and Lewis (1991) for male college students.

Cooper (1992) proposes that event-level studies of sexual risk-taking and alcohol use might let us assess issues of casual order – that is, whether alcohol disinhibition leads to high-risk sex, or whether sexual intentions or fears lead to alcohol use. After reviewing several time-link studies which differ on their findings about the existence of an event-specific association between alcohol and high-risk sex, she suggests that alcohol use may be more likely to be related to risky sex (a) among adolescents and (b) for the first intercourse between two partners.

Alcohol Use and Drug Injection: Many youth who are infected with HIV, HBV, and other parenterally-and-sexually-transmissible pathogens have been infected through drug injection. Thus, it is important to understand the relationships between alcohol use levels and becoming a drug injector. Unfortunately, little is known about the etiology of drug injection. The large cross-sectional and longitudinal studies of drug use among youth have either not asked about it or have found that too few subjects report injecting drugs to analyze. Even data on heroin use are beset by problems of small numbers of cases and, indeed, of probable considerable inaccuracy or undercounting (Denise Kandel, personal communication, December 29, 1993).

Models of adolescent progression to drug use have suggested that legal drugs like alcohol and cigarettes might function as gateway drugs, followed by marijuana as a second stage in the progression, with very few youth going on to harder drugs without using the gateway drugs. Kandel *et al.* (1992) found that such progression holds for alcohol or cigarettes, marijuana, other illicit drugs, and finally medically prescribed drugs in a cohort followed from ages 15 to 35. (As mentioned, their data set does not allow separate analysis of heroin use.) Early age of first use of a substance and high frequency of use of that substance were strong predictors of progression to a higher stage. Alcohol was the key first-level gateway drug for males, but for females use of either cigarettes or alcohol sufficed to progression to marijuana use.

In a study of 12th graders in New York, Kandel and Yamaguchi (1993) found that crack smoking (which has been linked to high-risk sex and thence to HIV and STDs {Chiasson *et al.* 1991} could also be fit into a stage model, with the initial stage for males being alcohol use and for females cigarette use, followed by marijuana, intranasal cocaine, and finally crack. Subjects who went on to crack use were characterized by having earlier ages of onset of alcohol use, of cigarette use, of marijuana use, and of intranasal cocaine use than those who did not use crack.

Johnson (1988) also found that a stage model applied, with intensive marijuana use being a precursor to progression to using other drugs even among youth who were drinking large amounts of alcohol. Nonetheless, alcohol intoxication was a predictor of progression to other drugs such as cocaine. In a study we conducted of heroin sniffers' progression to injection, intensity of non-injected drug use was a significant predictor of injecting drugs during follow-up (Des Jarlais *et al.*, 1992).

In sum, despite the lack of prior research on the causes of drug injection, it seems likely that heavy alcohol use in early adolescence is a first important step on the way to the later use of cocaine or heroin. Most drug injectors, thus, pass through stages in which they are heavy drinkers and/or users of gateway drugs. Such stages in drug use progression, however, are not immutable and, given the relative legality and availability of various drugs, as well as the historical and cultural context of drug use in different societies, other trajectories of drug use may occur. Thus, many heavy users of alcohol do not go on to using marijuana, and even fewer go on to using cocaine or heroin. Other forces, including the social networks with which youth interact and also youths' personalities and biographies, also seem to affect who becomes a drug injector.

Drug and Alcohol Use and Social Networks: Little research has been done on the social networks of problematic alcohol users. There has been some research on the social networks of alcoholics in treatment (Bloomfield, 1990; Favazza & Thompson, 1984) or focused on whether the networks of problem drinkers are heavily composed of other problem drinkers and whether this reinforces their drinking behaviour (Skog 1990). Social learning theories of alcohol use have found that the members of social networks influence drinking behaviours (Falk *et al.*, 1982), although the way in which such influence operates depends on the relationships to social network members and to the situations in which it is exerted (Kandel *et al.*, 1978; White *et al.*, 1991). Among peers, the association between subjects' alcohol use patterns and their peers' patterns seems to be a reciprocal product of both social influence and differential association (Downs 1987; Kandel, 1985; Gorman & White, in press), although peer influence on adolescent substance use may be stronger for females than for males and for whites than for African Americans (Farrell & Danish, 1993; Kandel, 1985). Unfortunately, research on the social networks of youthful alcohol drinkers or of youthful users of gateway drugs has not yet focused on the probability that other network members would actually be infected with HIV or other agents, nor on whether they would be behaviourally prone to such infection (due to drug-injecting or particularly high-risk sex behaviours), nor on whether peers' risky sexual behaviours would influence subjects' sexual behaviours. Nevertheless, given evidence that such problem behaviours as heavy alcohol use, drug use, delinquency and precocious sexual behaviour are associated with each other (Jessor & Jessor, 1977; White, 1992), it seems likely that the peer groups of many adolescent problem drinkers will include drug injectors, crack smokers, and others who engage in large amounts of high-risk sex.

Research on the social networks of drug injectors has examined factors such as drug injecting and sexual behaviours within networks, and the potential and actual consequences of this for HIV transmission (Friedman *et al.*, 1993; Friedman *et al.*, in press(a); Klovdahl *et al.*, 1994; Neaigus *et al.*, 1993; Potterat, 1992). Much research is needed on the extent to which network factors influence infection with HIV or other sexually – or parenterally – transmitted pathogens, and also on the extent to which network factors affect high-risk behaviours.

Predictors of Problem Substance Use and Other Problem Behaviours

In contrast, there is a vast literature on the predictors of alcohol and drug "abuse" among youth. Many of these predictors have also been identified as predictors of delinquency, "precocious" sexual behaviour, and other behaviours that are frowned upon by the authorities (which are thus often called "problem behaviours".) Further, although little research has been conducted among youth that has focused on the predictors of unsafe sex or of injecting with potentially infected syringes or drug mixtures, current knowledge suggests that many of the predictors of problem behaviours are also predictors of these direct risk factors for parenterally – and sexually – transmitted diseases. Below, we discuss some of these common predictors.

Personal Characteristics and Risk

Early conduct disorder and antisocial behaviour have been identified as predictors of alcohol/drug use in adolescence (White, 1992) as well as of adult alcoholism (Hesselbrock *et al.*, 1985; Rutter, 1992; Zucker & Gomberg, 1986). Similarly, engaging in antisocial behaviours predicted high risk sexual behaviour among adolescents in grades 8 through 12 in Oregon (Biglan *et al.*, 1990). Stiffman *et al.* (1992) found that conduct disorder (as well as depression and anxiety) is a predictor of AIDS risk behaviours among youth. In addition to antisocial personality, tendencies towards impulsivity, general risk taking, and sensation seeking have been associated with alcohol and drug use in adolescence (Bates *et al.* 1986; Jaccard & Wilson, 1991; Zuckerman, 1979). This same risk-taking profile has been associated with precocious sexual behaviour (White & Johnson, 1988).

Sexual abuse and other severe trauma during childhood or adolescence are also risk factors for HIV and STD infection and for behaviours such as alcohol/drug use, early sexual activities, and prostitution (Bayatpour *et al.*, 1992; Brown & Finkelhor 1986; Fullilove *et al.*, 1992; Paone *et al.*, 1992). For example, Gutman *et al.*, (1991) found that of 96 HIV-positive children, 14 had evidence of having been sexually abused. Vermund *et al.*, (1990), in a study of adolescents in a New York City detention facility, found that both boys and girls who were infected with gonorrhea or syphilis were more likely to report a history of sexual abuse than those who were not infected. Amaro *et al.*, (1989) found that, among a sample of adolescent mothers, drug users were more likely to have reported 'negative life events' such as being physically threatened or abused. In our ethnographic interviews with female drug injectors and commercial sex workers in Bushwick, many reported that they had been abused sexually when they were young. They also said that this was one reason why they began to use drugs. In contrast, although Dembo *et al.*, (1992) found that sexual victimization is related to marijuana/hashish use and other criminal behaviours, they did not find it to be related to alcohol use. Yet studies of women in alcohol treatment indicate high rates of sexual abuse (Wilsnack & Wilsnack, 1993).

Interpersonal Factors that Influence Gateway Substance Use and Sexual and Drug Risk Behaviours

Peer influence is a factor that affects whether youth begin to drink alcohol, the age at which drinking starts, and the amounts and situations in which it occurs (White *et al.*, 1991). One specific form which peer influence can take is when friends offer an adolescent a psychoactive substance to use; this was a very strong predictor of early adolescent use of gateway drugs (alcohol, cigarettes, marijuana) in a study of 7th and 8th graders (Ellickson & Hays, 1992). Peers can also influence sexual risk behaviour among adolescents. Billy *et al.* (1984, 1986) found that adolescent females who have sexually active best friends are more likely to become sexually active (while adolescent males were more likely to select best friends on the basis of sexual experience). Walter *et al.* (1992) found that students whose friends had intercourse with no (or inconsistent) use of condoms were much more likely to engage in high-risk sexual or drug behaviours. The role of peer pressure and support in influencing HIV risk behaviours and risk reduction among drug injectors is also well established in the literature (Abdul-Quader *et al.*, 1990; Huang *et al.*, 1989; McKeganey & Barnard, 1992), whereas maintaining social ties with non-injecting family members and friends seems to be associated with injecting in less risky ways (Neaigus *et al.*, 1994).

One mechanism through which peer influence may operate is through individual perceptions of group characteristics. Studies on condom use and acceptance highlight the role of perceptions of peer group norms and behaviours (Leland & Barth, 1992). DiClemente (1992) found that sexually active adolescents who perceived peer norms as supporting condom use were more likely to use condoms consistently. Adolescents' condom use has been associated with their perceptions of their sexual partners' insistence on or willingness to use them (Pendergast *et al.*, 1992).

The structure and functioning of the family during childhood and adolescence affect alcohol and drug use and sexual behaviour. (Dornbusch, 1989 and White *et al.*, 1991 review research on the relationship between family factors and risky behaviour.) The best predictors of youthful drinking habits are parents' attitudes and behaviours toward alcohol use (Barnes, 1977). In fact, most research suggests that parents who drink teach their children to drink. Thus, drinking behaviour, including heavy drinking, is the result of socialization experience in the family (White *et al.*, 1991). In addition, the quality of the interaction between adolescents and their parents and the quality of the home environment have been shown to influence adolescents' drinking regardless of what the parents' habitual use may be. Positive family relationships, attachment to family, communication, discipline, conflict, parental love, parental control, and family management techniques have significant influences (Glynn, 1981; Kandel *et al.*, 1978; White *et al.*, 1991). These same variables affect adolescent drug use (Gorman & White, in press). Likewise, family background variables, including the personality and child-rearing practices of the parents, are strongly related to later problem drinking and alcoholism in the offspring (Barnes, 1977; White *et al.*, 1991). Siblings' alcohol and drug use patterns are significant shapers of drug use and perhaps alcohol use (Clayton & Lacy, 1982; Needle *et al.*, 1986).

Hofferth *et al.* (1987) found that the age at which adolescent females initiate sexual activity is associated with the age at which their mothers initiated intercourse, and that adolescents with mothers or siblings who became pregnant during their teens were also more likely to become pregnant as teenagers. Studies of family structure have shown that adolescents in single parent households are more likely to initiate sexual activity earlier (Dornbusch, 1989; DuRant *et al.*, 1990; Franklin, 1988). Family emotional stability, as indicated by either a close relationship between the adolescent and a parent, or by a harmonious atmosphere in the home, has been shown to be protective against several types of risk behaviour. Conversely, emotional instability (such as parental discord or divorce) and physical instability (e.g., making many residential moves) are predictors of several risk behaviours. Coercive authority relationships between parents and children may increase youths' risk behaviours (Biglan *et al.*, 1990; Dornbusch, 1989).

Literature reviews and contemporary studies indicate that family history of parental alcoholism and/or problem use strongly influence drinking patterns and other problem outcomes of offspring (Pandina & Johnson, 1989, 1990). Most studies find that parental alcohol abuse is associated with impaired social functioning in children, including higher levels of interpersonal conflict, impaired problem solving techniques, and lower levels of family cohesion (Jarmas & Kazak, 1992). Subjects with a family history parental alcoholism, as well as children of heavy drinking parents, report high level of anxiety, stress, depression and an undercontrolled behavioural style (aggressiveness, rebelliousness, impulsivity) which may manifest itself also as delinquent behaviour (Johnson & Pandina, 1991; Mann *et al.*, 1987; Rolf *et al.*, 1988; Tarter *et al.*, 1990). Subjects with a family history of parental alcoholism have also been found to exhibit low level of social orientation, self-efficacy and goal directedness. (See Russell *et al.*, 1985, for a review). The manifestations of these factors contribute to a complex array of risk factors for subsequent outcomes including precocious sexual behaviour, antisocial behaviour and criminal behaviour in addition to adult alcoholism (Johnson & Tiegel, 1991; Sher, 1991).

Factors related to relationships with peers and with the structure and functioning of the family may be related to one another. Those who are susceptible to peer influence may be more likely to have weak bonds to their families, which may stem from a history of troubled family relationships. At the same time, those with strong social ties to members of their peer group and who may be more influenced by them, may further weaken their ties to their families. The developmental interaction between the structure and functioning of the family and the influence of peer relationships may be an important determinant of later problem behaviours, such as intense and precocious use of alcohol and other drugs.

Sociodemographic Factors in Substance Use, Risk Behaviours, High-Risk Networks, and Infection

Sociodemographic characteristics, such as social class, race/ethnicity, and gender have been associated with alcohol use, risk behaviours, and infections. Social class is directly related to drinking and heavy drinking (Clark & Hilton, 1991), but appears to be inversely related to alcoholism (Helzer, 1991). Thus, although "upper" class persons are more likely to drink than lower class ones (and 'what' they drink and the circumstances of their drinking patterns may differ), among drinkers alcoholism is higher among those of "lower" class. Alcoholism and heavy drinking are higher among males than females (Clark & Hilton, 1991; Helzer, 1991). Black 8th, 10th and 12th grade students report less drinking and less heavy drinking than whites or Hispanics (Johnston *et al.*, 1993), and among adults abstention is higher among blacks than whites or Hispanics (Caetano, 1991). Among white and Hispanic women, but not among black women, single and younger women are more likely to have alcohol problems (Caetano, 1991).

Homelessness is also tied to high-risk behaviours and networks. Homeless youth often engage in commercial sex work (including same-sex sex) in order to survive. They use alcohol and drugs to self-medicate against physical discomfort, loneliness and psychological distress, and some of them turn to injecting their drugs. As a consequence, they have high rates of STDs and of HIV infection (Bowler *et al.*, 1992; Clatts, Davis & Sotheran, 1994; Rotheram-Borus *et al.*, 1994).

Gender may also involve biological factors that can influence the probability of infection. Female and minority adolescents are particularly at risk of HIV infection (Rotheram-Borus & Koopman, 1991). The sociobehavioural patterns, however, are complex. In a national probability sample, Catania *et al.* (1992) found that males were more likely to report having multiple sexual partners, but that woman were more likely to have a high-risk primary sexual partner. Aral *et al.*, (1991), similarly, find that men aged 18 and 19 are more likely to report having had more than one sex partner in the preceding year. Women, persons with low education, blacks, and Hispanic women are more likely to be infected with HSV-2 in a San Francisco neighbourhood (Siegel *et al.*, 1992); and blacks, women, older persons, previously named persons, poorer persons, and urban residents were more likely to be infected with HSV-2 in the second NHANES (Johnson *et al.*, 1989). Black, Hispanic and Native Americans have a higher incidence of STDs than do whites (Aral *et al.* 1991), and blacks and Hispanics (particularly Puerto Ricans) are disproportionately likely to have AIDS or HIV (Friedman *et al.*, 1987; Selik *et al.*, 1988, 1989) This may be due to greater frequencies of high-risk behaviour – Marmor *et al.*, (1987) found this to explain higher HIV seroprevalence among black drug injectors – or it may be due to different patterns of changing partners or of getting medical care for treatable STDs. Holmbeck *et al.* (1990) found that lower socioeconomic status is related to being sexually active and to presenting with an STD among black women aged 12-20; and lower income is associated with infection with HSV-2 (Breinig *et al.* 1990; Johnson *et al.* 1989).

Social patterns make sexual (and drug injection) contact more frequent within racial/ethnic groups than between them. Thus, if an infectious agent is more prevalent in a given racial/ethnic group, each risky act by a member of that group will be more likely to be conducted with an infectious partner – and thus more likely to lead to infection. For example, black women do not report riskier sexual behaviour than white women, but nonetheless have higher STD rates (Aral *et al.*, 1991). This pattern probably is one cause of the findings by Hahn *et al.* (1989) that race remains a significant predictor of STD morbidity even with socioeconomic status controlled.

RECENT FINDINGS ON THE SEXUAL NETWORKS OF ADOLESCENTS

In this section, we report on several studies of the sexual networks of adolescents. Such risk networks are pathways through which HIV and other infectious agents can spread. To the extent that they are social networks, they also can be pathways for social influence.

The first of these studies starts with a sample of drug injectors of various ages, and allows us to describe the non-injecting youth with whom they have sexual relationships. These other studies are, first, additional preliminary data from the study of youth aged 18-21 in Bushwick that was discussed above (with infection rates presented in Table 2); and, secondly, data from a network study of young adolescents in Atlanta and San Juan.

In the Social Factors and HIV Risk study (which, as has been discussed above, was conducted in Bushwick, a major drug-injection and drug sales neighbourhood in New York City), 767 IDUs provided us with a data about 617 of their sexual relationships. As has been elsewhere reported (Goldstein *et al.*, 1995), comparisons of the self-reports of drug injectors and the descriptions their network members gave of their relationships and of each other provide strong evidence that the behavioral and relationship data collected in this study are accurate. Almost half (299) of the sexual relationships reported by the IDUs in this study were with persons who do not inject drugs. Further, few (23) of these relationships were with non-IDUs who were 21 years old or younger, with the youngest non-IDU sex partners being three 16 years-olds. In 8 of these 23 relationships (including one longstanding Lesbian relationship between two women), the drug injector was infected with HIV. One seropositive male IDU who was 24 years old had sexual relations with 5 different young women; a 17 year old and an 18 year old with each of whom he had been having sex for two years, a 19 year old with whom he had been having sex for 6 years, and two 20 year olds with whom he had been having sex for one and for four years, respectively. He reported that he always used condoms with four of these women; for the fifth of his relationships, no data are available. Indeed, in 14 out of 21 (67%) of the relationships for which HIV data are available, the drug injector who was the research participant reported that she or he always used condoms. There were no instances in which an HIV-infected IDU reported having unprotected sex with any of these non-injecting youth (nor with other non-injectors aged 25 years or less, although there were some instances of unprotected sex in relationships of HIV+IDUs with older non-injectors.)

These data provide a number of reasons for optimism. Although data are not available about the HIV serostatuses of the non-IDU sex partners (since they were not themselves participants in the research), it is notable that few youthful (aged 21 or below) non-IDUs seem to be at high risk of HIV transmission from this group of almost 800 IDUs. That is, only 23 are reported to be having sex with these 767 IDUs (although this may well be an underestimate since research subjects may have reported on fewer relationships than they really had in order to shorten their interviews). Although 36% of these non-IDU youth are having sex with HIV-infected IDUs, consistent condom use seems to be taking place in most if not all of these relationships.

Furthermore, this study also suggests that the average age at which people start to inject drugs has been increasing during the AIDS epidemic. Among long-term injectors (those who began to inject 7 or more years before they were interviewed for the study), their average age of initiation was 19; but among new injectors, the average age of initiation has increased to 27. This may imply that, as time goes on in an AIDS epidemic, fewer people begin to inject drugs, and that they do so later in life. This, in turn, would probably decrease the number of adolescents who have sexual relations with IDUs.

We have recently begun to collect data from a representative household sample of Bushwick 18-21 year olds. So far, data have been analyzed for 65 of these youth. None of them are infected with HIV, hepatitis C, or HTLV-I or HTLV-II, and only two youth have been infected with hepatitis B. Furthermore, none of them reports ever having injected drugs, or ever having had sex with anyone whom they know has injected drugs. Although these data are from a small number of youth, and thus must be regarded as preliminary, they tend to support the implications of the Social Factors and HIV Risk study – the youth in this potentially high-risk neighborhood seem to have fewer high-risk contacts with IDUs than might have been expected.

On the other hand, most of these youths have lives that are still quite fluid in that they have not settled down to the prototypical working class or middle class life style with a settled job and/or spouse. Thus, only 12% are living with a spouse, and 55% are living with parents and/or step-parents. Almost half (46%) were neither employed nor in school at the time of interview. Twenty-three percent report having sold drugs at least once in their life (and 13% have done so in the last year). Violence has been an important part of their lives: approximately 10% report having been physically abused by a police officer, 30% have been threatened or stabbed with a knife, 27% have been caught in a random shoot-out, 22% have been threatened or shot at with a gun, 33% have been mugged or robbed with a threat of violence, and 14% of the women and 5% of the men report having been sexually abused. Over half (51%) report having carried a weapon such as a knife, club or gun. Almost half (48%) report having been subjected to racial or ethnic discrimination, and 24% of the women report having been subjected to gender discrimination. In the socioeconomic context of a minority community with widespread unemployment and a world economy that is unlikely to provide even

Table 3
Percents Reporting Initiating Drug Use and Sexual Activity in Given Age Ranges in Initial Probability Samples in Atlanta and San Juan

	Percent Initiating			
	Atlanta		San Juan	
Age Category	Drugs (N*)	Sex (N*)	Drugs (N*)	Sex (N*)
Less than 12	0% (43)	7% (43)	0% (52)	6% (52)
12-13 years	0% (43)	18% (40)	6% (52)	19% (48)
14-15 years	4% (25)	17% (17)	17% (23)	24% (17)

*N is the denominator used to calculate the percentages. It excludes those who have not reached the age category and those who initiated the behavior prior to the age category.

moderate-paying or moderate-stability jobs, and in the context of widespread drug injection and other drug use by older persons, many of these youth are at high risk of themselves becoming drug injectors or the sex partners either of drug injectors or the sex partners of drug injectors.

Data are also available for the age of initiation of illicit drug use, injecting drug use, and sexual activity from studies in high-risk neighborhoods of African American young adolescents in Atlanta, Georgia and of young Puerto Ricans in San Juan, Puerto Rico. At each site, a probability sample of 12-15 year olds living in a specified geographic area served as generators of a network sample via a random-walk procedure.

The proportions initiating these activities among the 43 Atlanta youth and 52 San Juan youth in the initial probability samples are given in Table 3. For these individuals, the overall estimate of the proportions of those reporting drug use, drug injecting, and sexual activity were 2.3% (standard error = 2.1%), 0.0%, and 30.2% (standard error = 5.1%) in Atlanta and 13.5% (standard error = 4.8%), 0.0% and 30.8% (standard error = 6.5%) in San Juan.

Table 4
Percents of Network Respondents Reporting Initiating Drug Use and Sexual Activity in Given Age Ranges in Total Samples in Atlanta and San Juan

	Percent Initiating			
	Atlanta		San Juan	
Age Category	Drugs (N*)	Sex (N*)	Drugs (N*)	Sex (N*)
Less than 12	0% (129)	11% (129)	0% (143)	6% (143)
12-13 years	0.7% (127)	14% (113)	4% (143)	13% (134)
14-15 years	5% (83)	29% (63)	14% (84)	21% (68)
16-18 years	21% (38)	70% (20)	8% (39)	41% (32)
19-29 years	0% (12)	–	0% (18)	–

*N is the denominator used to calculate the percentages. It excludes those who have not reached the age category and those who initiated the behavior prior to the age category.

The random-walk procedure (4-node, 3-step) generated 129 unique respondents in Atlanta and 143 in San Juan. All named associates between the ages of 12 and 29 were eligible for selection as respondents. The proportions initiating sex and drug use at each age for all respondents of that age or above are shown in Table 4.

The potential for exposure related to injecting drug use to HIV in this population of adolescents was examined in two ways; direct drug injecting experience and having sex with a drug injector. No subjects reported injecting drugs themselves, and none reported having sex with a known drug injector, in either Atlanta or San Juan.

CONCLUSIONS

As discussed above the causes of the use of gateway drugs are quite complex. Contributing causes may include genetic factors (Goodwin, 1985), family socialization, psychological problems, sexual abuse or other trauma, general problem behavior, peer socialization, or other factors. Many of these causes may also lead to high-risk sexual or drug injecting behaviors, to involvement in high-risk social networks (via differential association), and/or to infection with HIV or other sexually – or parenterally-transmitted pathogens.

There are a number of important unresolved issues about youth and how their lives may put them at risk for HIV and other infections. Some of the most important issues that need more research include:

(1) The prevalence of infections (particularly HIV) among youth in high-risk communities and (2) the extent to which involvement in high-risk networks affects the probability of infection with each infectious agent. Much is known about the risk behaviors that can lead to becoming infected, but much less in known about the extent to which social network factors mediate infection. It is likely that pathogens that are less prevalent (Friedman *et al.,* 1995), and those with a lower probability of transmission in a given sexual or drug injection event, are more subject to network effects.

The preliminary data from the Bushwick youth study provide some encouragement. Although the confidence limits are wide due to the small number of observations, the observed levels of infections suggest that the heterosexual diffusion of HIV and other infections from IDUs to youth may be quite limited. (On the other hand, if the true rates of infection are at the upper bounds of the confidence limits for HIV, HCV, HTLV-I and HTLV-II, rates of more than 4% of youth in a neighborhood being infected with potentially fatally diseases would be quite alarming.) Even the hepatitis B rate, at 3.4%, is less than had been expected – although it may suggest a danger if, as these youth grow older, their malleable social condition (as indicated by the high percents who lack jobs, who have not yet established their own homes but instead live with their parents or grandparents, and who deal drugs) may lead them into drug-injecting or into sexual relations with drug injectors or the partners of drug injectors.

The data from the Bushwick studies of youth and of drug injectors, and those from the studies of youth in Atlanta and San Juan, suggest some reasons why there is little diffusion of HIV and other infections from drug injectors to the youth of these communities. Few youth are having sex with drug injectors (although many older non-IDUs do have sex with IDUs in Bushwick), and in most cases those IDUs they do have sex with have been injecting for relatively few years and thus may be less likely to have become infected with HIV yet (Friedman *et al.*, 1989; Jose *et al.*, 1993). Furthermore, at least in Bushwick, when youth do have sex with (infected) IDUs, the transmission of HIV and other infections is often prevented by condom use. The limited extent of sex between youthful non-IDUs and IDUs is likely to be a function of: (a) the extent to which sex partnerships in a community tend to be between people of similar age; (b) the age at which IDUs begin to inject drugs – which in New York, at least, has increased considerably; and, perhaps, (3) the extent to which fear of AIDS and/or stigmatization of drug injectors deter the formation of IDU/non–IDU sexual partnerships.

(3) In sum, then, these data suggest that the greatest HIV threat which non-IDU heterosexual youth in the United States, and perhaps in other economically developed countries, face may be the possibility that they will themselves begin to inject drugs or that, in their 20's or 30's, they will engage in non-injected use of crack cocaine, heroin or other drugs that will put them at risk of forming sexual partnerships with drug injectors. Thus, further research is clearly needed on the causal pathways and influences that lead some youth in a high-risk community to: (a) engage in problem drinking or use of gateway drugs; (b) become drug injectors; (c) engage in high frequencies of unprotected sex; (d) and thus, perhaps, to have high-risk drug or sex partners and (e) to become infected with HIV or other pathogens.

Implications for Prevention

Even though there is a lot that is not yet known about how adolescents come to be at risk for HIV infection, HIV and other serious diseases are spreading among them. Thus, it seems valuable to list some possible approaches to prevention that might be effective.

These will be discussed in terms of the unit of intervention (that is, what is the "target" of the intervention); and will sometimes involve consideration of the nature of the actor (i.e., who intervenes).

All such programs need to include recognition of developmental probabilities: Many youth who do not engage in sex or in problem drinking at age 12 will do so by age 14; and many who have no friends who use hard drugs at age 14 will have many who do so by age 16. Thus, training and discussions need to be based on the fact that youth, as they grow up, are "moving targets" in "moving social environments," and thus that issues that are not problematic (and, perhaps, not of interest) at one age will be dilemmas or risks a year or two later.

Individual as target of the intervention

Education is needed on HIV and STDs; sex; drugs; on how to analyze interpersonal and social structural situations, the risks they may pose, and the opportunities they provide for effective individual or group action.

Targeted programmes can help users of "gateway" drugs not to move on to using "harder" drugs; and help smokers and snorters of heroin and/or cocaine not to progress to injecting.

Skills training programmes can be effective. These should include risk avoidance; condom negotiations; and how to function effectively in peer pressure situations.

Medical interventions can also help stem the spread of HIV. Controlling STDs among adolescents both removes physical morbidity in the genitals that can facilitate HIV transmission, and provides an opportunity for education targeted at youth who may be at particularly high risk. Youth who can benefit from it should have easy access to drug abuse treatment. Counseling should be available for those whose history or personality make them susceptible to becoming drug injectors. An example of such a group is the large number of youth who have been sexually abused at some time in their lives.

Family as target of the intervention:

To the extent that they are effective, programmes that prevent sexual and physical abuse in the family will reduce the number of youth who grow up particularly susceptible to becoming drug injectors. Similarly, special prevention efforts should be developed for youth whose parents or older siblings engage in high-risk behaviors.

Peer groups as target of the intervention:

Help adolescents form groups against AIDS.

Conduct group discussions of how to support each other to reduce risk.

Potentially infectious groups as target of the intervention.

Work with IDUs, and with adolescents with STDs, to help mobilize their efforts to protect others.

Socioeconomic environment as target of the intervention:

Drug injecting seems to be more frequent among persons of the working class, and within the working class, among those in its least well paid and most-often unemployed sections. Since few sexual partnerships cross social class or status lines, this means, in turn, that persons in these groups are particularly likely to have sex with partners who are infected with HIV or other agents that can be transmitted by infected syringes. Similarly, members of subordinated racial/ethnic groups, such as African Americans or Puerto Ricans in New York, seem to be at increased risk of AIDS and STDs.

This suggests that programmes should be developed to improve the situations of poor people and of subordinated racial/ethnic groups.

Even more, it suggests that we need to develop ways to end poverty and racial subordination, and to create classless societies. Such needs are important in reducing the spread of HIV and other infectious diseases, and have their own inherent value as well. It would be naive, however, to think that such changes come easily. They require powerful social movements, such as Polish Solidarity in 1981, the movement among African Americans in the 1960s, and that among French workers in 1968. One issue to be considered, and perhaps a strategy to be pursued, is to find ways whereby existing and future group efforts to prevent the spread of HIV and/or to deal with policy and care issues that affect those who have been infected can contribute to the building of wider social movements.

It is worth keeping in mind, however, that none of the movements mentioned above attained all of its goals. Indeed, in each case, partial goal attainment has not prevented the development of new forms of major social ills such as increased use of injected drugs among (at least) African Americans and the Polish working class since 1970 and 1982, respectively. Thus, considerable creativity and discussion is needed.

ACKNOWLEDGEMENTS

We would like to acknowledge financial support from the National Institute of Allergy and Infections Diseases (grant A134723) and the National Institute of Mental Health (grant MH47649).

REFERENCES

Abdul-Quader, A., Tross, S. *et al.* (1990) Street-recruited intravenous drug users and sexual risk reduction in New York City. *AIDS* 4: 1075-1079.

Amaro, H., Zuckerman, B., Cabral, H. (1989). Drug use among adolescent mothers. *Pediatrics* 84: 144-151.

Aral, S.O., Schaffer, J.E., Mosher, W.D., Cates, M., Jr. (1988) Gonorrhea rates. *Am J Public Health* 78: 702-703.

Aral S.O., Fullilove, R.E., Coutinho, R.A., van den Hoek, J.A.R. (1991) Demographic and societal factors influencing risk behaviors. In: Wasserheit, J.N., Aral S.O, Holmes, K.K. (eds). (1991). *Research Issues in Human Behavior and Sexually Transmitted Diseases in the AIDS Era.* Washington, DC: Am. Society for Microbiology: 161-176.

Barnes, G.M., (1977) The development of adolescent drinking behavior: An evaluative review of the impact of the socialization process within the family. *Adolescence* 12: 571-591.

Bates, M.E., Labouvie, E.W., White, H.R. (1986) The effect of sensation-seeking needs on changes in drug use during adolescence. *Bull of Soc of Psychologists in Addict Behav* 5: 29-36.

Bayatpour, M., Wells, R.D., Holford, S. (1992) Physical and sexual abuse as predictors of substance use and suicide among pregnant teenagers. *J Adolescent Health* **13**: 128-132.

Bell, T.A., Hein, K. (1984) Adolescents and sexually transmitted diseases. In: Holmes K, *et al.* (eds), *Sexually Transmitted Diseases.* New York: McGraw Hill International Book Co.: 73-84.

Biglan, A., Metzler, C.W. *et al.* (1990) Social and behavioral factors associated with high-risk sexual behavior among adolescents. *J Behav Med* **13**: 245-261.

Billy, J.O.G., Rodgers, J.L., Udry, J.R. (1984) Adolescent sexual behaviour and friendship choice, *Social Forces* **62**: 663-678.

Billy, J.O.G., Udry, J.R. (1986) The influence of male and female best friends on adolescent sexual behavior. *Adolescence* **20**: 21-31.

Bloomfield, K.A. (1990) *Community In Recovery.* Doctoral dissertation, Public Health, Univ. of California.

Bolton, R., Vincke, J., Mark, R., Dennehy, E., (1992) Alcohol and risky sex. *Med Anthro* **14**: 323-363.

Bowler, S., Sheon, A.R., D'Angelo, L.J., Vermund, S.H. (1992) HIV and AIDS among adolescents in the United States: Increasing risk in the 1990s. *J Adolescence* **15**: 345-371.

Breinig, Kingsley, *et al.* (1990) Epidemiology of genital herpes in Pittsburgh. *J Infect Dis* **162**: 299-305.

Brown, A., Finkelhor, D. (1986) Impact of child sexual abuse. *Psychol Bull* **1**: 66-99.

Burke, D.S., Brundage, J.F. *et al.* (1990) Human immunodeficiency virus infections in teenagers. *JAMA* 263:2074-2077.

Caetano, R. (1991) Findings from the 1984 national survey of alcohol use among US Hispanics. In: Clark W.B., Hilton M.E. (eds.), *Alcohol in America.* New York: State University of New York Press: 293-307

Catania, J.A., Coates, T.J. *et al.* (1992) Prevalence of AIDS-related risk factors and condom use in the United States, *Science* **258**: 1101-1106.

Centers for Disease Control. (1991) Premarital sexual experience among adolescent women – United States, 1970-1988. *MMWR* **39**: 929-932.

Centers for Disease Control. (1992) Summary of notifiable diseases, United States 1991. *MMWR* **40**: 11.

CDC. (1994) *HIV/AIDS Surveillance: U.S. AIDS cases reported through June 1994.* Atlanta: CDC.

Chiasson, M.A., Stoneburner, R.L. *et al.* (1991) Heterosexual transmission of HIV-1 associated with the use of smokable freebase cocaine (crack). *AIDS* **5**: 1121-1126.

Clapper, R.L., Lewis, P. (1991) A retrospective study of risk-taking and alcohol-mediated unprotected intercourse. *J Subst Abuse* **3**: 91-96.

Clark, W.B., Hilton, M.E. (1991) *Alcohol in America.* New York: State University of New York Press.

Clatts, M.C., Davis, W.R., Sotheran, J.L. (1994) At the cross-roads of HIV infection: A demographic and behavioral profile of street youth in New York City. Presented at Second Annual Symposium on Drug Abuse, Sexual Risk and AIDS: Prevention Research 1995-2000. Flagstaff, Arizona.

Clayton, R.R., Lacy, W.B. (1982) Interpersonal influences on male drug use and drug use intentions. *Int J Addict* **17**: 655-66.

Cooper, M.L. (1992) Alcohol and increased behavioural risk for AIDS. *A/c Health Research World* **16**: 64-72.

DeHovitz, J.A., Zenilman, J. *et al.* (1992) The prevalence of herpes simplex type II

(HSV-2) antibody in a cohort of inner-city women. 8th Int. Conf. on AIDS, Amsterdam {poster PoC 4650}.

Dembo, R., Williams, L., Wothke, W., Schmeidler, J., Brown, C. (1992) The role of family factors, physical abuse and sexual victimization experiences in high-risk youth's alcohol and other drug use and delinquency. *Violence and Victims* 7 (No. 3): 245-266.

Denzin, N.K. (1987) *The Alcoholic Self.* Beverly Hills, CA: Sage.

Des Jarlais, D.C., Casriel, C., Friedman, S.R., Rosenblum, A. (1992) AIDS and the transition to illicit drug injection, *Br J Addict* 87: 493-498.

DHHS (1991) *Healthy People 2000.* Washington, DC: U.S. Department of Health and Human Services. DHHS Publication No. (PHS) 91-50212.

DiClemente, R.J. (1992) Psychosocial determinants of condom use among adolescents. In: DiClemente R.J. (ed.), *Adolescents and AIDS: A Generation in Jeopardy.* Newbury Park, CA: Sage: 34-51.

Dornbusch, S.M. (1989) The Sociology of adolescence. *Ann Rev Sociol* **15**: 233-259.

Downs, W.R. (1987) A panel study of normative structure adolescent alcohol use and peer alcohol use. *J Studies Alc* **48**: 167-175.

DuRant, R.H. Pendergrast, R. Seymore, C. (1990) Sexual behavior among Hispanic female adolescents in the United States. *Pediatrics* **85**: 1051-1058.

Ellickson, P.L. Hays, R.D. (1992) On becoming involved with drugs. *Health Psych* **11**: 377-385.

Ericksen, K.P. Trocki, K.F. (1992) Behavioral risk factors for sexually transmitted diseases in American households. *Soc Sci & Med* **34**: 843-853.

Falk, JL, Schuster, C.R. Bigelow, G.E., Woods, J.H. (1982) Progress and needs in the experimental analysis of drug and alcohol dependence. *Am Psych* **37**: 1124-1127.

Farrell A.D., Danish, S.J. (1993) Peer drug associations and emotional restraint *J Consult Clin Psych* **61**: 327-334.

Favazza, A.R., Thompson, J.J. (1984) Social networks of alcoholics. *Alc: Clin & Exper Res* **8**: 915.

Franklin, D.L. (1988) Race, class and adolescent pregnancy. *Am J. Orthopsychiat* **58**: 339-354.

Friedman, S.R., Sotheran, J.L., *et al.* (1987). The AIDS epidemic among Blacks and Hispanics. *Milbank Quarterly* **65**: 455-499.

Friedman, S.R., Rosenblum, A., Goldsmith, D.S. *et al.* (1989) Risk factors for HIV-1 infection among street-recruited intravenous drug users in New York City. 5th Int. Conf. on AIDS, Montreal, Canada (abstract T.A.O. 12).

Friedman, S.R., Jose, B., Neaigus, A., *et al.* (1993) Female injecting drug users get infected sooner than males. 9th Int. Conf. on AIDS, Berlin (PO-DO3-3512).

Friedman, S.R., Jose, B., *et al.* (1994) Consistent condom use in relationships between seropositive injecting drug users and sex partners who do not inject drugs. *AIDS.* **8**: 357-361.

Friedman, S.R., Neaigus, A., *et al.* (in press) Network and sociohistorical approaches to the HIV epidemic among drug injectors. In: Catalan, J., Sherr, L., Hedge B., (Eds)., (1997) The Impact of AIDS: Psychological and Social Aspects of HIV infection. Chur, Switzerland: Harwood Academic Publishers.

Friedman, S.R., Jose, B., Deren, S., Des Jarlais, D.C., Neaigus, A., National AIDS Research Consortium, (1995) Risk factors for HIV seroconversion among out-of-treatment drug injectors in high and low-seroprevalence cities. *Am J Epidemiol.* **142:** 864-874.

Fullilove, M.T., Lown, E.A., Fullilove, R.E. (1992) Crack 'hos and skeezers: Traumatic experiences of women crack users. *J Sex Research* **29**: 275-287.

Gayle, H.D., D'Angelo, L.J. (1991) Epidemiology of acquired immunodeficiency syndrome and human immunodeficiency virus infection in adolescents. *Pediat Infec Dis J* **10**: 322-328.

Geschwender, J.A. (1978) *Racial Stratification in America.* Dubuque, IA: Wm. C. Brown Co.

Gillmore, M.R., Butler, S.S. Lohr, M.J., Gilchrist, L. (1992) Substance use and other factors associated with risky sexual behavior among pregnant adolescents. *Fam Plan Persp* **24**: 255-261, 268.

Glynn, T.J. (1981) From family to peer. In Lettieri, D.J., Ludford, J.P. (Eds.) *Drug Abuse and the American Adolescent.* Washington: US Government Printing Office. NIDA Monograph #38.

Goldstein, M.F., Friedman, S.R. *et al.* (1995) Self-reports of HIV risk behavior by injecting drug users: Are they reliable? *Addiction.* **90**: 1097-1104.

Goodwin, D.W. (1985) Genetic determinants of alcoholism. In: Mendelson JH, Mello NK (eds.), *The Diagnosis and Treatment Of Alcoholism* (2d ed.). New York: McGraw-Hill: pp 65-87.

Gorbach, S., Bartlett, J., Blacklow, N. (Eds.), (1993) *Infectious Diseases.* Philadelphia: WB Saunders.

Gorman, D.M. & White, H.R. (in press) You can choose your friends, but do they choose your crime? Implications of differential association theories for crime prevention policy. Barlow, H. (Ed.). *Criminology and Public Policy: Putting Theory to Work.* Boulder, CO: Westview Press.

Gutman, L.T., St. Claire, K.K., Weedy, C. *et al.* (1991) Human immunodeficiency virus transmission by child sexual abuse. *Am J Dis Child* **145**: 137-141.

Hahn, R.A., Magder L.S., Aral, S.O., Johnson, R.E. Larsen, S.A. (1989) Race and the prevalence of syphilis infections in the US population. *Am J Public Health* **79**: 467-470.

Helzer, J.G. (1991) Demographics of alcohol use and misuse. International Symposium on Alcohol, Society and the Determinants of Health. Kiawah Island, SC.

Hesselbrock, V.M., Hesselbrock, M.N., Stabeneau, J.R. (1985) Alcoholism in men patients subtyped by family history and antisocial personality. *Journal of Studies on Alcohol* **46**: 59-64.

Hofferth, S.L., Kahn, J.R., Baldwin, W. (1987) Premarital sexual activity among U.S. teenage women over the past three decades. *Fam Plan Persp* **19**: 46-53.

Holmbeck, G.N., Waters K.A., Brookman, R.R. (1990). Psychosocial correlates of sexually transmitted diseases and sexual activity in black adolescent females. *J Adolescent Res* **5**: 431-448.

Hook,E.W. III, Cannon, R.O., Nahmias, A.J. *et al.* (1992a) Herpes simplex virus infection as a risk factor for human immunodeficiency virus infection in heterosexuals. *J Infect Dis* **165**: 251-255.

Hook, E.W. III, Reichart, C.A., Upchurch D.M., Ray, P., Celentano, D., Quinn, T.C. (1992b) Comparative behavioral epidemiology of gonoccal and chlamydial infections among patients attending a Baltimore, Maryland, cosexually transmitted disease clinic. *Am J Epidemiol* **136**: 662-672.

Huang, K.H.C., Watters, J.K., Case, P. (1989) Compliance with AIDS prevention measures among intravenous drug users. 5th Int. Conf. on AIDS, Montreal {M.D.O.5}

Jaccard, J., Wilson. T. (1991) Personality factors influencing risk behaviors. In: Wasserheit J.N. *et al.*, op. cit.: 177-197.

Jarmas, A.L., Kazak, A.E. (1992) Young adult children of alcoholic fathers. *J Clin Psych* **60**: 244-251.

Jessor, R., Jessor, S. (1977) *Problem Behavior and Psychosocial Development: A Longitudinal Study of Youth.* New York: Academic Press.

Johnson, J., Tiegel, S. (1991) Treating adults raised by alcoholic parents. *Recent Devel Alc* **9**: 347-359.

Johnson, R.E., Nahmias, A.J., Magder, L.S. *et al.* (1989) A seroepidemiologic survey of the prevalence of herpes simplex virus type 2 infection in the United States. *N Engl J Med* **321**: 7-12.

Johnson, V. (1988) A longitudinal assessment of predominant patterns of drug use among adolescents and young adults. In: Chesher, G., *et al.* (Eds.), *Proceedings of the Melbourne Symposium on Cannabis.* Canberra: ANCADA, Australian Department of Health.

Johnson, V., Pandina, R.J. (1991) Familial and personal drinking histories and measures of competence in youth. *Addict Behav* **16**: 453-465.

Johnston, L.D., O'Malley, P.M., Bachman, J.G. (1993). *National Survey Results on Drug Use from the Monitoring the Future Study, 1975-1992.* Rockville, MD: US Department of Health and Human Services.

Jones, R.B., Wasserheit, J.N. (1991) Introduction to the biology and natural history of sexually transmitted diseases. In: Wasserheit, J.N. *et al.*, op. cit.: 11-37.

Jose, B., Friedman, S.R., Neaigus, A. *et al.* (1993). Syringe-mediated drug-sharing (backloading). *AIDS* 7: 1653-60.

Kandel, D.B. (1985) On the process of peer influences in adolescent drug use. *Adv Alc Subst Abuse* **4**: 139-163.

Kandel, D.B., Kesler, R.C., Margulies, R.S. (1978) Antecedents of adolescent initiation into stages of drug use. In: Kandel D (Ed.), *Longitudinal Research into Drug Use.* Washington: Hemisphere-Wiley: 73-99.

Kandel, D.B., Yamaguchi, K., Chen, K. (1992) Stages of progression in drug involvement from adolescence to adulthood. *J Studies Alc* **53**: 447-457.

Kandel, D.B., Yamaguchi, K. (1993). From beer to crack. *Am J Public Health* **83**: 851-855.

Keller, S.E., Bartlett, J.A., Schleifer, J., Johnson, R.L. (1991) HIV-relevant sexual behaviour among a healthy inner-city heterosexual adolescent population in an endemic area of HIV. *J Adoles Health* **12**: 44-48.

Kipke, M., Futterman, D., Hein, K. (1990) HIV infection and AIDS during adolescence. *Medical Clinics of North America* **74**: 1149-1166.

Klassen, A.D., Wilsnack, SC. (1986) Sexual experience and drinking among women in a U.S. national survey. *Arch Sex Behav* **15**: 363-392.

Klovdahl A.S., Potterat, J.J. *et al* (1994) Social networks and infectious disease. *Soc Sci Med* **38**: 79-88.

Leigh, B.C. (1990) The relationship of substance use during sex to high-risk sexual behavior. *J Sex Res* **27**: 199-213.

Leland, N.L., Barth, R. (1992) Gender differences in knowledge, intentions and behaviors concerning pregnancy and sexually transmitted disease prevention among adolescents. *J Adoles Health* **13**: 589-599.

Mann, L.M., Chassin, L., Sher, K.J. (1987) Alcohol expectancies and the risk for alcoholism. *J Consult Clin Psych* **55**: 411-417.

Martin, J.L., Hasin, D.S. (1990) Drinking, alcoholism and sexual behavior in a cohort of gay men. *Drugs & Society* **5**: 49-67.

McKeganey, N., Barnard, M. (1992) *AIDS, Drugs and Sexual Risk.* Buckingham, UK: Open University Press.

Neaigus, A., Friedman, S.R., Curtis, R. *et al.* (1994) The relevance of drug injectors' social networks and risk networks for understanding and preventing HIV infection. *Soc Sci Med* **38**: 67-78.

Neaigus, A., Friedman, S.R. *et al.* (1995). Using dyadic data for a network analysis of HIV infection and risk behaviours among injecting drug users.

Needle, R.H., Coyle, S.L., Genser, S.G. & Trotter, R.T. (Eds.) *Social Networks Drug Abuse and HIV Transmission* (NIDA Research Monograph ISI). Rockville, MD: National Institute on Drug Abuse. PP. 20-37.

Needle, R., McCubbin, H., Wilson, M. *et al.* (1986) Interpersonal influences in adolescent drug use. *Int J Addict* **21**: 739-766.

O'Leary, A., Goodhart, F., Jemmott, L.S., Boccher-Lattimore, D. (1992) Predictors of safer sex on the college campus. *J Am College Health* **40**: 254-263.

Padian, N., Shibosky, S.C., Hitchcock, P.J. (1991) Risk factors for acquisition of sexually transmitted diseases and development of complications. In Wasserheit *et al*, op cit., pp. 83-96.

Pandina, R.J., Johnson, V. (1989) Familial drinking history as a predictor of alcohol and drug consumption among adolescent children. *J Studies Alc* **50**: 245-253.

Pandina, R.J., Johnson, V. (1990) Serious alcohol and drug problems among adolescents with a family history of alcoholism. *J Studies Alc* **51**: 278-282.

Paone, D., Chavkin, W., Willets, I., Friedmann, P., Des Jarlais, D.C. (1992) The impact of sexual abuse. Implications for drug treatment. *J Women's Health* **1**: 149-153.

Pendergast, R.A., DuRant R.H., Gaillard, G.L. (1992) Attitudinal and behavioral correlates of condom use in urban adolescent males. *J Adoles Health* **13**: 133-139.

Potterat, J.J. (1992). "Socio-geographic space" and sexually transmissible diseases in the 1990s. *Today's Life Sci* Dec.: 16-22, 31.

Rolf, J.E., Johnson, J.L., Israel, E., Baldwin, J. Chandra A. (1988) Depressive affect in school-aged children of alcoholics. *Br J Addict* **83**: 841-848.

Rotheram-Borus, M.J. Koopman, C. (1991) HIV and adolescents. *J Primary Prevent* **12**: 65-82.

Rotheram-Borus, M.J., Feldman, J., Rosario, M., Dunne, E. (1994). Preventing HIV among runaways. In DiClemente, R.J. & Peterson, J.L. (Eds.), *Preventing AIDS*. New York & London: Plenum. 175-188.

Russell, M., Henderson, C., Blume, S. (1985) *Children of alcoholics: A review of the literature.* New York: Children of Alcoholics Foundation, Inc.

Rutter, M. (1992). Adolescence as transition period: Continuities and discontinuities in conduct disorder. *J of Adolescent Health* **13**: 451-460.

Schoenbaum, E.E., Stern, L.S., Webber, M., Drucker, E., Gayle, H. (1989) HIV antibody and high risk behaviors among non-intravenous drug using women obtaining abortions in the South Bronx, New York City. 5th Int. Conf. on AIDS, Montreal, Canada {abstract Th. D.P.1}.

Selik, R.M., Castro, K.G., Pappaioanou, M., Buehler, J.W. (1989) Birthplace and the risk of AIDS among Hispanics in the United States. *Am J Public Health* **79**: 836-839.

Selik, R.M., Castro, K.G., Pappaioanou, M. (1988) Racial/ethnic differences in the risk of AIDS in the United States. *Am J Public Health* **78**: 1539-1545.

Shafer, M.A. Hilton J.F., *et al.* (1993) Relationship between drug use and sexual behaviors and the occurrence of sexually transmitted diseases among high-risk male youth. *Sex Trans Dis* **20**: 307-313.

Sher, K. (1991) Psychological characteristics of COA. *Recent Devel Alc* **9**: 301-326.

Siegel, D., Golden E. *et al.* (1992) Prevalence and correlates of herpes simplex infections: The population-based AIDS in Multiethnic Neighborhoods study. *JAMA* **268**: 1702-1708.

Skog, O-J. (1990) Alcohol in a social network perspective. *Alcologia* **2**: 13-21.

Stiffman, A.R., Dore, P., Earls, F., Cunningham, R. (1992) The influence of mental health problems on AIDS-related risk behaviors in young adults. *J Nerv Ment Dis* 180: 314-320.

Stinson, F.S., DeBakey, S.F., Grant, B.F., Dawson, D.A. (1992) Association of alcohol problems with risk for AIDS in the 1988 National Health Interview Study. *Alcohol Health & Res World* **16**: 245-252.

Strunin, L., Hingson R. (1992) Alcohol, drugs, and adolescent sexual behavior. *Int J Addictions* **27**: 129-146.

Tarter R.E., Kabene, M., Escallier, E.A. Laird, S.B., Jacob, T. (1990) Temperament deviation and risk for alcoholism. *Alc: Clin & Exper Res* **14**: 380-382.

Temple, M.T., Leigh, B.C. (1992) Alcohol consumption and unsafe sexual behavior in discrete events. *J Sex Res* **29**: 207-219.

Vermund, S.H., Alaxander-Rodriguez, T., Macleod, S., Kelley, K.G. (1990). History of sexual abuse in incarcerated adolescents with gonorrhea or syphilis. *J Adoles Health Care* **11**: 449-452.

Walter, H.J., Vaughan, R.D. *et al.* (1992) Factors associated with AIDS risk behaviors among high school students in an AIDS epicenter. *Am J Public Health* **82**: 528-532.

White, H.R. (1992) Early problem behavior and later drug problems. *J Res Crime Deling* **29**: 412-429.

White, H.R., Johnson, V. (1988) Risk taking as a predictor of adolescent sexual activity and use of contraception. *J Adoles Res* 4: 317-31.

White, H.R., Bates, M.E., Johnson, V. (1991) Learning to drink. In: Pittman DJ, White HR (Eds.), *Society, Culture and Drinking Patterns Reexamined.* New Brunswick: Rutgers Center of Alcohol Studies: 177-197.

Wilsnack, S., Wilsnack, R. (1993) Epidemiologic research on women's drinking. In: Gomberg E.S.L., Nirenberg TD (Eds.), *Women and Substance Abuse.* Norwood, NJ: Ablex Publishing: 62-99.

Zelnick, M., Kantner, J., Ford, K. (1981) *Sex and Pregnancy in Adolescence.* Beverly Hills: Sage.

Zucker, R.A., Gomberg, E.L. (1986) Etiology of alcoholism reconsidered. *Am Psych* **41**: 783-793.

Zuckerman, M. (1979) *Sensation Seeking.* Hillsdale, NJ: Lawrence Erlbaum Associates, Inc.

9

Adolescents and Emerging Sexuality

GLYNIS M. BREAKWELL

INTRODUCTION

This chapter explores emerging sexuality among adolescents. It aims to provide a review and overview of current studies, concepts and knowledge. This is an important prerequisite to any understanding of sexuality or sexual risk on the light of HIV and AIDS and should form the backdrop against which prevention, intervention, knowledge and skill based learning approaches are introduced to this population. The chapter sets out to explore studies on sexuality, psychological and social meanings of sexual activity and issues such as menarche onset, the lexicon of sexuality, sexual identities and sexual preoccupations. Gender differences are also explored together with notions of sexual self efficacy, risk taking and vulnerability. As this chapter provides some background understanding, the reader should look to some of the applications of these notions in chapters 4-7 where applications to HIV and the impact of AIDS on adolescents is explored in greater depth.

EMERGING OR CONTINUING?

There is now reasonably consistent evidence that there is no sexual moratorium or period of latency during late childhood such as that postulated by Freud. From a study of childhood sexuality involving interviews with over 800 children in Australia, North America, Britain, and Sweden, Goldman and Goldman (1982) concluded that children aged five to fifteen years of age were increasingly interested in exploring sexual topics in linear progression with age. Cross-cultural studies over the last forty years have shown that so long as a society is not repressive toward childhood sexual activity, such behaviour continues and may even become more frequent during the preadolescent years. Certainly, the Kinsey studies (Kinsey *et al.*, 1953) illustrated that sexual experimentation does not even slow down during this period.

Of course, the psychological and social meaning of sexual activity during the early years of adolescence changes in parallel with the physical maturation that occurs during this period. The first sign of puberty in girls is usually the beginning of breast development, which may occur as early as 8 years of age or as late as age 13. This is closely followed by the appearance of pubic hair, the lengthening of the vagina and the enlarging of the uterus. Menarche usually occurs as breast growth nears completion but its onset is influenced by socio-economic factors, heredity, family size, and nutrition. Irregular menstrual cycles are common in the first year after menarche and ovulation does not usually occur but vaginal secretions, not always tied to sexual excitation, are likely to increase. In boys, puberty usually starts about two years later than in girls. The first change entails the growth of testes stimulated by increased testosterone production, which also initiates the growth of the penis, prostate, seminal vesicles and epididymis. Before puberty, ejaculation is impossible because the prostate and seminal vesicles do not function until they receive the appropriate hormonal cues. In Western societies, boys start genital development at 11-12 years of age and the genitals reach adult size between age 14 and 15. The amount of time required for genital development varies between individuals and is sometimes only one year but sometimes 5.5 years. Sperm production only becomes fully established during puberty, and it is only then that fertility is achieved. Growth of pubic hair is coterminous with genital development and is usually followed 1-2 years later by facial and axillary hair. Testosterone stimulation of the larynx causes it to grow and results in the voice "breaking" and deepening.

These physical and hormonal changes prime the adolescent for a broader range of sexual activities. They provide the necessary equipment but do not determine how it will be used. There is little evidence that would argue that hormonal levels predispose sexual orientation, though there is some suggestion that those who undergo pubertal changes earlier do tend to be both more sexually active and active at a younger age whether in relation to auto-eroticism or intercourse with others.

THE LEXICON OF SEXUALITY

Socio-cultural context shapes the forms that sexuality can take; determining what is acceptable at what ages. Even before the adolescent has completed the physical transformations of puberty, the social meaning of each element of these changes will have been communicated to him or her with more or less clarity and success. Acquiring the lexicon of sexuality is a major task of adolescence. While sexual activity may develop continuously throughout childhood, it takes on a different social significance after puberty largely because thereafter sexuality can lead to conception.

Adolescents are faced with the task of assimilating, ordering and decoding the often conflicting messages which they will receive about sex and sexuality. Their difficulties are magnified because so much of what society has to say about sex and sexuality is either ambiguous or treated as a series of secrets to be uncovered. The facts are obfuscated with ill-defined emotional overtones which subvert any simple acquisition of the vocabulary and grammar of sexuality. If you listen to older adolescents talking about how they first learned about eroticism (as distinct from the biology of sexual reproduction) you realise that there are no easily available or authoritative manuals that define what all new participants need to know. At least, this is true in most cultures and, even where formal sexual initiation ceremonies still exist, the introduction is usually partial.

Actually producing any simple guidance about sexuality for adolescents would not be easy. It is made difficult because what is considered normal sexuality in one culture will be shunned in another. What is regarded as acceptable sexuality changes over time even within the same culture. This is evidenced clearly in the last fifty years in the systematic increases in the percentage of people who report having had sexual intercourse before the age of sixteen and before marriage. Details of the changing pattern of sexual behaviour have been presented in an earlier chapter. Mostly, these statistics are derived from surveys which rely upon retrospective self-reports of behaviour. Of course, it may be that changes in the norms which control willingness to report some behaviours actually explain some of the apparent changes in sexual behaviour. Perhaps people are now just more willing to admit that they had sexual intercourse before they were sixteen or before they get married. Yet even this reflects a modification in what is considered acceptable sexuality. The willingness to admit to having had sex at a young age, for instance, is itself a product in part of the revision of dominant codes of sexuality. Adolescents have to cope with learning these changing codes and, within them, with constructing a sexual identity for themselves appropriate for their imminent adulthood.

SEXUAL IDENTITIES

Sexuality is more than simply a repertoire of sexual desires and behaviours. It is enmeshed in complex systems of beliefs about the broader roles of men and women and their relationships with each other. Individuals have differential access to these systems of belief depending upon their socio-economic status, ethnicity, religion, nationality, and so on. Frequently, they will be aware of a number of different ideologies of sexuality. The lack of any single clear societal prescription concerning sexuality offers the adolescent some latitude of freedom in the construction of a personal sexual identity.

Adolescence is often regarded by psychologists and sociologists as a period of turmoil and uncertainty but it is also, perhaps as a consequence, a time of increasing freedom and autonomy. This independence is sometimes believed to be expressed in so-called "sexual rebellion": a rejection of the perceived societal expectations, particularly of family or church, usually associated with promiscuity or risk-taking. However, the empirical evidence for large scale rebellion is not strong. In fact, within any one culture, idiosyncratic patterns of either behaviour or belief are rare. For the majority even sexual experimentation follows a predictable routine, that followed by the majority of one's peers. Changes in patterns of sexual behaviour and belief are actually gradual, resembling evolution rather than rebellion, and tend to involve many people. Few adolescents capitalise individually on the possibilities for creativity in the construction of sexual identity which undoubtedly do potentially exist.

This rejection of sexual individuality during adolescence can be explained in terms of general identity processes. A major motive force in the construction of adolescent identities is the need to gain acceptance from peer groups (and from society more generally) by avoiding manifestations of uniqueness or difference. In relation to sexual identity this motive yields remarkable similarities across adolescents in the way they perceive themselves and in the way they characterise what is typical for men and women in general. Breakwell (1994) reports the findings of a longitudinal study of the sexual beliefs and activities of 16-21 year olds in the UK conducted between 1989 and 1993. As part of this research, Breakwell elicited from respondents their social representations of differences between male and female sexuality: several hundred young men and women were asked to describe on a series of fourteen characteristics what they believed to be appropriate behaviour for a man and for a woman in sexual relationships. Analyses of their responses showed that males and females tended to agree remarkably well about the female sexual role but to disagree about the male role in sexual relationships. They tend to agree that the female role is expected to be sensitive, passive, responsible for contraception, romantic, and faithful. They are also expected to be less willing to have premarital sex and more likely to merely pretend to enjoy sex. When it comes to the representation of male sexuality, men and women disagree. Women are more likely to say that men are keen on sexual experimentation, exploitative of their partners, and ignorant when it comes to eroticism. Men represent the male role as seductive and controlling of when and how sex occurs. Of course, both images are consistent with traditional stereotypes of male sexuality which has been portrayed as recreational, narcissistic, insensitive, exploitative, oriented towards immediate gratification, grasping of every sexual opportunity, and lacking real feeling for the partner (Farrell, 1975; Simon and Gagnon, 1983; Tiefer, 1987; Bolton and MacEachron, 1988; Seidler, 1989; Gross, 1978; Brod, 1990).

It is interesting to examine how far beliefs about these general images of sex differences in sexuality are linked to individual sexual behaviour. To explore the relationship between the social representations and actual sexual behaviour, Breakwell attempted to identify whether there were any subgroups within her sample that held marked different representations. Her analyses revealed that there were two very clear subgroups in the female sample that held consistently different views about the sexuality of women. One group, about one third of the sample, essentially saw women as less interested in sex, more lacking control of when sex occurs, more sexually passive, more likely to avoid sexual experimentation, and more unwilling to have premarital sex. The two groups differed in their views about most aspects of female sexuality but these areas comprise their fundamental disagreement. The startling finding, however, was that the members of the group which generally regarded the female sexual role as passive were clear in their rejection of this role for themselves. They stated that they would not themselves behave in the passive fashion that they thought was characteristic of women in general. In fact, members of this group were actually more likely to have started to have sex at a younger age, to have had more sexual partners, and to be less likely to use condoms. These data reveal a fascinating paradox: for women in adolescence, believing that the expected role of women in sexual relationships is passive or inhibited is associated not only with the rejection of that role but also with more risky patterns of behaviour. Looking at this from the other direction: the young women who thought that the expected sexual role of women was more exploitative, experimental and seductive, were more likely to accept that role for themselves but were then less likely to be sexually active in any way, and, when they were, their behaviour was more constrained.

These data suggest that amongst young women, at least in the UK in the late 1980s-early 1990s, there were two dominant views of female sexuality. These can be broadly caricatured as the active and the passive. While adherence to the active representation is very much tied to the individual's concept of herself as a sexual being, it does not predict behaviour during adolescence. It may, of course, be linked to behaviour plans or expectations and actual behaviour later. In contrast, adherence to the passive representation is dissociated from the individual's sexual self concept and this is reflected in behaviour during adolescence. These findings indicate that all adolescent women certainly do not simply internalise and act upon what they perceive to be commonly accepted norms of female sexuality. Nor do they all simply reject these norms in the general throes of adolescent rebellion. In fact, what seems to be happening is, firstly, that different subgroups believe different norms to be operative, and, secondly, within those subgroups, there are similar behavioural reactions. So far, the origins (perhaps in socio-economic, religious, familial influences) of these sub-groupings have not been identified and there is no evidence that the young women who share belief and behaviour patterns in this way are actually directly aware of each others' existence.

Interestingly, when the male respondents in the Breakwell study were examined, it was found that they fell into two roughly equally-sized subgroups in terms of the beliefs they held about male sexuality. These subgroups were differentiated largely in terms of the extent to which they regarded men as being "sexually responsible" (i.e. sensitive, faithful, not exploitative, and so on) (Breakwell & Millward, in press). Those who identified men as sexually responsible were more likely to identify with this and to be relatively sexually cautious (that is, they had less sexual partners, followed safer sexual practices, and had begun their sexual activity at a later age). Conversely, those who regarded men generally as sexually irresponsible were less likely to identify themselves with such a role but they were more likely to be relatively sexually uninhibited. It seems, then, that for young men the representation they have of what is typical of male sexuality is quite influential in predicting their own behaviour, even when notionally they claim that they are different from what they believe to be the "typical man".

These data suggest that adolescent males are less likely than adolescent females to reject or ignore their social representations of acceptable forms of gendered sexuality in making their own decisions about their own behaviour. The finding emphasises that it is necessary when thinking about adolescent sexuality and the influences which shape it to model its development in males and females separately. Young men and young women share many of the same sexual socializing influences (for example, the media, literature, and so on) but their receptivity to them has been differentially sensitised by the time that they reach adolescence. Of course, the messages from these sources are different but, even were they the same, it is unlikely that young men and women would respond to them identically.

SEXUAL PREOCCUPATIONS

A common component of popular beliefs about adolescence is that it is a period typified by preoccupation with sex and sexuality. It is assumed that adolescents are driven, if not obsessed, by the need to know more about sexuality: what people can do and what they will do, with whom, when, where and how often. Such sexual curiosity may not be assumed to be linked directly to seeking out personal sexual experience but it is assumed to be tied to the shaping and tuning of sexual desire. However, the evidence available only partially supports these popular assumptions. Curiosity about sexuality characterises early adolescence (in Western industrialised communities 10-12 years of age) but is soon satisfied. By mid-adolescence most will claim to know a lot about sexuality and certainly most will claim to know enough. Whether this "knowledge" is accurate or adequate is questionable. Quizzes meant to test sexual knowledge given to teenagers regularly reveal misunderstandings not simply on such topics as conception and contraception but also on matters concerning sexual arousal. Even though their sexual knowledge may actually be flawed, the fact they feel that they know enough means that manifestations of sexual curiosity fade quickly in adolescence. At least, few admit to their ignorance and fewer admit to being curious.

Sexual preoccupation during adolescence in fact seems to have more to do with sexual yearning than sexual curiosity. This yearning starts with just wanting sexual encounters. These are effectively unspecific wants since the partner is not identified and the sex acts desired are hazy. From this, the next phase in sexual yearning develops. This entails much more detailing in imagination of the encounter or series of encounters: the first contact, the seduction scene, the consummation, and so on. What is then wanted, yearned for, is this specific imagined sexual experience. According to the accounts of some interviewees in the Breakwell study, these imagined sexual encounters can be elaborated over several years and, indeed, form the basis for their adult sexual fantasies. Of course, the type of sexual encounter which is yearned for may never be experienced in reality.

The disparity between the imagined and the actual experiences of sex during adolescence seems in some to heighten the yearning but in others to subdue it. The nature of the relationship between sexual imagination and sexual action is not understood. In some situations, imaginations drives action but, in others, it clearly becomes a substitute for it. Adolescents imagining sexuality can be said to be mentally practising routines that they might use later. They can equally well be said to be suppressing possible sexual action by focusing upon sex in their imaginations. In fact, however, there is no strong evidence that sexual fantasies are less frequent, detailed or vivid when individuals are more sexually active. This leads to the conclusion that sexual imagination and sexual action have no inevitable or predictable relationship.

Males are commonly thought to be more preoccupied than females with sexuality during adolescence. This gender difference is often overstated and oversimplified. Gender differences undoubtedly interact with socio-economic class, cultural, and educational differences in predicting sexual preoccupations. Even if one focuses purely upon the gender differences the situation is not simple. Males, on average, may be recognisably more preoccupied with the mechanics of sexuality but females, on average, are more preoccupied with the relationships within which they see sexuality to be lodged. Young women are more likely (again on average) to be preoccupied with ideas of romance than young men. Adolescent women often have well-formulated systems of belief about what is romantic and how sex and romance should be brought together. Notably, typically these romantic beliefs tie sex to faithfulness. At least in mid-adolescence, females are concerned with establishing a relationship which is romantic and "steady". Sexuality is virtually always seen by adolescent women in the context of such a faithful relationship. Young men may be more preoccupied with sexuality for its own sake, young women are concerned with sexuality as a component of becoming part of a couple. These systems of belief can lead some young women to feel sexually insecure because they have not achieved the ideal romantic attachment by some deadline assumed by them and their peers to be appropriate.

Of course, sexual insecurity is experienced by both males and females at this age. While preoccupation with sexuality per se may be limited, concern about sexual attractiveness is widespread. Both sexes become more concerned with body image as they enter adolescence. Deviation from the cultural norm in any aspect of appearance can be a cause for anxiety. Most find strategies for coping with what they initially perceive as their disadvantages in the sexual stakes (Breakwell, 1986). For instance, as people move through adolescence the standards they apply when judging physical appearance become less severe and less restrictive; more variations become acceptable – including themselves. Another strategy involves revising the overall significance of physical attraction when judging people so that other aspects are taken into account such as intellect or character – usually some aspect on which they can also score better. Even by the end of adolescence, however, some will still feel that they are not sexually attractive by their own standards. These sometimes compensate by minimising the importance of sexuality in their concepts of themselves. Alternatively, they may set about affirming their personal attractiveness by becoming involved in a series of short-term but intense affairs.

Given all of these factors which determine the shape of sexual preoccupations, it is not possible to say how long such preoccupations persist in adolescence. It is tempting to suppose that preoccupation declines as experience increases and curiosity, fantasies, and the need to be found attractive are satisfied. It seems possible that sexual nonchalance, even boredom, replaces preoccupation at some point in late adolescence as confidence develops and surprises become infrequent. Unfortunately, there is no reliable evidence on this as yet.

SEXUAL SELF-EFFICACY

Bandura introduced the concept of self-efficacy (1977). He postulated that people's perceptions of their own capabilities influence how they act, their motivational levels, their thought patterns, and their emotional reactions to demanding situations. Self-efficacy is high when the individual believes that he or she can perform an act or complete a task. It is low when failure or inability is anticipated. Self-efficacy has nothing to do with outcome of the behaviour. It is purely to do with whether people believe that they could behave in a particular manner. In keeping with social learning theory, expectations about self-efficacy are supposed to be derived from three sources of information: past performance; observation of the performance of others; and feedback from others about one's capacity. Additionally, where positive emotional arousal occurs, self-efficacy may be generally raised. Self-efficacy in a particular area of activity is initially determined by experiences of success or failure but subsequently it influences our choices of activities and environments. People normally choose activities and environments in which they feel they are self-efficacious.

Bandura's theory is concerned with specific self-efficacy as it relates to particular activities or tasks. This allows for someone to be highly efficacious in some things but low in others and moderate in many. Breakwell, in the study introduced above, examined sexual self-efficacy in adolescents. Sexual self-efficacy relates to the person's perception of his or her own ability to perform appropriately in sexual encounters and relationships. What is deemed appropriate will differ across individuals and this is not important. What matters is the individual's own estimate of how far he or she is capable of meeting the demands of the sexual situation. Sexual self-efficacy is not a property of performance which can be objectively assessed. It is a subjective reaction to the possibility of performance and, subsequently, a reflection of performance in retrospect.

Adolescents vary markedly in their levels of sexual self-efficacy and, while efficacy levels generally increase with age, maturation does not eliminate individual differences. Some people remain lower in sexual self-efficacy throughout their early adulthood.

Sexual self-efficacy seems to be a significant influence upon behaviour. For instance, Breakwell, Millward and Fife-Schaw (1994) report that sexual self-efficacy is a factor in determining whether an individual who is motivated to practice safer sex (due to concerns about the risk of infection or as a result of normative pressure) will actually do so. People who have higher levels of sexual self-efficacy are more likely to carry out their intentions when it comes to the actual sexual encounter. It seems that self-efficacy in sexuality is intimately related to perceiving oneself to be in control. This sense of control encompasses choice of partner, choice of behaviours, and what could be called the "rules of engagement" (i.e. when and where sex takes place). Not surprisingly, sexual self-efficacy is associated with greater assertiveness in relationships. However, it is not related to levels of risk-taking. Some adolescents who are high on the sexual self-efficacy measures are very cautious, others are sexual gamblers.

There is no simple gender difference in sexual self-efficacy. Males and females do not, on average, differ in levels of sexual self-efficacy in those adolescent samples studied so far. The origins of sexual self-efficacy in experience, feedback and observation would suggest that there should be greater variation within males and within females than there is between them and this is indeed the case.

This efficacy dimension of sexuality does seem to have been overlooked until now and merits further exploration. It may be an important ingredient in shaping many decisions concerning sexuality during adolescence. For instance, it may be possible that a certain level of sexual self-efficacy has to be reached before an individual will be willing to initiate sexual activity. If sexual self-efficacy is actually developed through positive feedback, it may help to explain why adolescents tend to start to engage in sexual acts in a discrete and predictable sequence. Having been successful at hand-holding, they may feel they can be successful at kissing. Having been successful at kissing, they may feel they could be successful at more intimate caressing. Iterative success may be required in a socially accepted sequence to evolve sexual self-efficacy.

Of course, sexual self-efficacy is also worth exploring further because it is connected to the inherent power relations which are part of sexuality. Any sexual encounter involves a negotiation of who will be in control and for how long. Sexual self-efficacy is evolved successively in the context of these power negotiations. There is little data available on sexual encounters between adolescents and adults (i.e. not in the context of sexual abuse) but it would be valuable to examine how such encounters affect the development of sexual self-efficacy. Generalisations about the emergence of adolescent sexuality take adolescent-adolescent relationships to be the norm (and indeed they are statistically so) but this may obscure other important types of encounter in determining the formation of sexual desires and patterns of behaviour.

SEXUAL RISK-TAKING AND VULNERABILITY

Despite the ideology of romance and faithfulness which surrounds adolescent views of hetero-sexuality, the reality is that committed long-term relationships are the exception rather than the norm. Much more often, for heterosexual relationships the pattern is of a series of short but intense partnerships. While the partnership lasts, it is typified by exclusivity or "faithfulness" which is highly prized. A departure from faithfulness by either party normally indicates the irreparable breakdown of the relationship and, most often, for the unfaithful party signifies the advent of the next "steady" relationship. Initially, in such "steady" partnerships, a couple will normally practice safer sex, using condoms to prevent both conception and the transmission of diseases and not having anal intercourse. Very quickly, however, safer sexual practices are abandoned or adhered to spasmodically.

The series of studies of sexual activity patterns which revealed this tendency to shift from partner to partner and to drop safer sex soon after establishing a partnership have been implicitly interpreted as suggesting that adolescents take more sexual risks than older age groups. This has led some theorists to try to explain why adolescents take greater sexual risks. Basically, it has been argued that adolescents do this because they are more likely to believe that they are not vulnerable to the hazards involved. Essentially, it is argued that adolescents feel some heightened sense of personal invulnerability. They think: it might happen to someone else but not to me. Such perceptions of invulnerability in adolescence are supposed by some to stem from adolescent egocentrism (i.e. the inability to view what happens from any other perspective than one's own based on one's own immediate experiences). Inexperience, relative to adults, would lead the adolescent to be ignorant of personally-relevant examples of negative consequences of the risky behaviours and thus to the conclusion that it was safe to do them.

This sort of explanation, however, may be premature. There may be nothing to explain. The evidence that adolescents are greater sexual risk-takers than older people is sketchy. Any comprehensive data on sexual risk-taking for, say, the 35-30 age group are notably absent. Also, there are other reasons to believe that adolescents would not be particularly more likely to take risks. Research on inferential and attributional biases indicates that people underestimate their own vulnerability to negative events. They also tend to underestimate their vulnerability when the cause of the outcome is perceived as being under their own control rather than being due to external factors outside their control. However, there is currently no evidence that adolescents are more prone to these biases than adults (Bell and Bell, 1993). Furthermore, there is no evidence that adolescents have higher levels of defensive denial (Fiske & Taylor, 1984) which is said to result in unrealistic optimism about the outcomes of risk-taking and can encourage greater risk-taking. It is possible that adolescents would take greater sexual risks if risk-taking was associated with dividends in terms of self-esteem. People do show an optimistic bias in estimating the effects of risk-taking if the risk enhances or maintains self-esteem. However, for this to be a good explanation for adolescents taking greater sexual risks than older groups, it would need to be confirmed that sexual risk-taking was more salient for self-esteem in adolescence than subsequently. This has not yet been established.

While one hesitates to dismiss lightly the widely-held belief that adolescents perceive sexual risks differently than do adults, research which compares directly the perceptions of vulnerability in adolescents and adults has not been conducted. In this situation, and without evidence that adolescents employ different heuristic rules to adults when estimating probabilities associated with risk outcomes, the claims that adolescents take greater sexual risks and do so because they feel invulnerable need to be treated with caution. Risk-taking may characterise the sexuality of adolescence but it may do so because it characterises sexuality at all ages to some extent.

This leads to a more general conclusion for this chapter. Examining the development of sexuality in adolescence serves to emphasise the continuities not jut with childhood but also into adulthood. The evolution of sexual identity, sexual self-efficacy and sexual imagination and desire are life-span developmental processes.

REFERENCES

Bandura, A. (1977) Self-efficacy: toward a unifying theory of behavior change. *Psychological Review*, **84**, 191-215.

Bell, N.J. & Bell, R.W. (Eds.) (1993) *Adolescent Risk Taking* Newbury Park, California: Sage Inc.

Bolton, F.G. & MacEachron, A.E. (1988) Adolescent male sexuality: a developmental perspective. *Journal of Adolescent Research*, **3**, 259-273.

Breakwell, G.M. (1986) *Coping with Threatened Identities* London: Methuen.

Breakwell, G.M. (1994) The Echo of Power. (The Myers Lecture 1993). *The Psychologist*, February, 65-72.

Breakwell, G.M. & Millward, L.J. (in press) Sexual Self-Concept and sexual risk-taking. *Journal of Adolescence Special Issue on Adolescent Health*, **19**.

Breakwell, G.M., Millward, L.J. & Fife-Schaw, C.R. (1994) Commitment to 'Safer' Sex as a Predictor of Condom Use amongst 16-20 Year Olds. *Journal of Applied Social Psychology*. **24**, 189-217.

Brod, H. (1990) *The making of masculinities* Boston: Allen & Unwin.

Farrell, W. (1975) *The Liberated Man* New York: Bantam Press.

Fiske, S.T. & Taylor, S.E. (1984) *Social Cognition* Reading, MA: Addison-Wesley.

Goldman, R. & Goldman, J. (1982) *Children's Sexual Thinking* London: Routledge and Kegan Paul.

Gross, A.E. (1978) The male role in sexual behaviour. *Journal of Social Issues*, **34**, 87-107.

Kinsey, A.C., Pomeroy, W.B., Martin, C.E. & Gebhard, P.H. (1953) *Sexual Behaviour in the Human Female* Philadelphia: W.B. Saunders.

Seidler, V.J. (1989) *Rediscovering masculinity: reason, language and sexuality* London: Routledge.

Simon, W. & Gagnon, J.H. (1983) Sexual scripts: permanence and change. *Archives of Sexual Behavior*. **15**: 97-120.

Tiefer, L. (1987) In pursuit of the perfect penis: the medicalisation of male sexuality. In M.S. Kimmel (Ed.) *Changing Men: New Directions in Research on Men and Masculinity* Newbury Park, California: Sage. 165-184.

10

Adolescents Facing AIDS and Hemophilia: Neuropsychological and Psychosocial Findings and Issues

STEPHEN R. HOOPER & J. KENNETH WHITT

INTRODUCTION

Approximately four percent of all diagnosed cases of Acquired Immunodeficiency Syndrome (AIDS) have included children with hemophilia, and the numbers climb to 31% when adolescents (i.e., ages 13 through 19 years) with hemophilia are included (Jason, Stehr-Green, Holman *et al.*, 1988). At one point, it was estimated that as many as 43% of all adolescent male cases of AIDS resulted from contaminated blood and blood-products for the treatment of hemophilia or coagulation disorders, one of the largest groups of adolescents with AIDS (Jason *et al.*, 1988).

Although transmission of HIV via this mode has been virtually eliminated through effective donor screening and heat treatments of blood products, thus eliminating the development of new cases of HIV infection via this mode, individuals with hemophilia treated before April 1985 were significantly at risk (Stehr-Green, Holman, Jason, & Evatt, 1988). It has been estimated that at least 75% of persons with severe hemophilia (i.e., factor VIII) treated during that time were exposed to HIV through the use of contaminated factor concentrate (Stehr-Green *et al.*, 1988). If they have survived, many of the children who were infected at that time via this mode are now well into their adolescence, and the adolescents affected are now young adults. Since adolescence generally represents the transition from childhood into adulthood, it generally shares risk factors indigenous to both younger and older populations. Consequently, the adolescent hemophilia AIDS population continues to present challenges to professionals across many different settings.

In tandem with many of the other chapters in this volume, this chapter addresses specific concerns pertinent to adolescents facing AIDS and hemophilia. In this chapter we provide an overview of the literature on what is known about the general functioning of adolescents with hemophilia and AIDS, with a particular focus on the neuropsychological and psychosocial findings procured to date. In addition, we discuss a number of key issues confronting professionals working with this population.

OVERVIEW OF CURRENT FINDINGS

Neuropsychological:

It has been reported that children and adolescents who are HIV seropositive can show a wide variety of neurological, neuropsychological, and neurodevelopmental impairments (e.g., Aylward, Butz, Hutton *et al.*, 1992; Levenson, Mellins, Zawadzki, Kairam, & Stein, 1992; Novello, Wise, Willoughby & Pizzo, 1989; Stover, Pequegnat, Huffman *et al.*, 1990). Although somewhat disputed (e.g., Tennison, Messenheimer, Ehle *et al.*, 1989), Scott (1988) noted that over 50% of all HIV-positive children eventually show some form of central nervous system deficit or dysfunction. More recently, Brouwers, van der Vlugt, Moss, Wolters, and Pizzo (1995) demonstrated an association between white matter changes on brain CT scans and selected neurobehavioral dysfunction in children with symptomatic HIV disease.

These observations received further support from Papola, Alvarez, and Cohen (1994) who observed that over half (54%) of their sample of children and adolescents with vertically infected HIV (n = 90), of whom about 31% met criteria for AIDS, were functioning within the 'borderline' to 'mentally retarded' range of intelligence. In addition, about 84% of their sample exhibited some form of developmental language impairment, 63% received some form of special education, and about one-quarter of the sample was diagnosed with Attention Deficit-Hyperactivity Disorder. Additionally, approximately 16% of the sample manifested emotional difficulties severe enough to warrant a psychiatric diagnosis. Most of these concerns reflected affective symptoms and tended to emerge around adolescence. Despite the significance of these findings, it should be noted that results such as these have been asserted largely for children who acquired HIV prenatally or perinatally, and that many of these studies do not employ control and/or appropriate comparison groups. Further, these findings have not been derived from individuals with hemophilia.

Perhaps one of the first published studies to address this concern was conducted by Whitt, Hooper, Tennison *et al.* (1993). In this longitudinal study, efforts were made to detect subtle, but objective neuropsychological deficits in a sample of 58 children and adolescents with severe hemophilia. These efforts also attempted to clarify the relationship between early involvement of the central nervous system and the progression of HIV in this sample.

Subjects. The sample was recruited from a large regional hemophilia center and divided into two groups: an HIV+ group (n = 25) and an HIV - group (n = 33). The average age at the time of the initial assessment was about 13 years, and about two-thirds of each group was Caucasian. At the time of the baseline evaluation, 68% of the HIV+ sample had CD4 counts < 500, one HIV+ subject was receiving antiretroviral drug therapy, and only two HIV+ subjects were symptomatic. None had been diagnosed with AIDS. Outside of socioeconomic status, as defined by maternal education, the groups did not differ in any of the basic demographic variables.

Procedures. Each of the subjects participated in an array of neurologic, neuropsychologic, neuroradiologic, and electrophysiologic measures at baseline. All of the procedures except the neurologic examination were conducted without information pertaining the individual's HIV status or the major hypotheses of the study. The HIV-seropositive group was evaluated every six months over the course of the study, while the HIV-seronegative groups was evaluated at yearly intervals. More specifically, the neuropsychologic test battery initially was designed to assess neurodevelopmental domains of functioning that were hypothesized to show the central nervous system effects of HIV infection. These domains included fine-motor, attention, language, visual processing, memory, and cognition. Criteria for test selection included (1) relevance to known natural history of AIDS, (2) adequate psychometric properties and availability of age-specific normative data on which to base conversion of raw data into standard scores, and (3) sufficient brevity to minimize undue fatigue. All of the selected measures are commonly used in neuropsychological evaluations of children and adolescents.

The Fine-Motor Domain comprised tests designed to detect the presence of any lateralized deficits, and to tap fine-motor speed and control, visual-motor speed, and visual-motor output. Tasks included manual finger tapping, grooved pegboard, WISC-R/WAIS-R Coding, and the Developmental Test of Visual-Motor Integration.

Tasks for the Attention Domain were selected in order to address issues of selective visual and auditory attention, impulsivity, performance consistency, distractibility, and impulsivity. These measures included the Gordon Diagnostic System (Vigilance Subtest), Goldman-Fristoe-Woodcock Auditory Selective Attention Test, Trail-Making Test (Parts A and B), and the Freedom from Distractibility Factor from the respective WISC-R or WAIS-R.

The Language Domain was comprised of measures selected to tap expressive and receptive abilities. Measures included the Peabody Picture Vocabulary Test, Sentence Repetition Test from the Detroit Test of Learning Aptitude, Goldman-Fristoe-Woodcock Auditory Discrimination Test, Controlled Oral Word Association (FAS), and the Verbal Comprehension Factor from the respective WISC-R or WAIS-R.

The Visual Procession Domain was constructed to measure a hierarchical array of Visual-perceptual functions including visual discrimination, visual-spatial abilities, and visual organization. Tasks included the Benton Judgment of Line Orientation

Test, Developmental Test of Visual-Motor Integration, and the Perceptual Organization Factor from the age-appropriate Wechsler Intelligence Scale.

Memory Domain tasks were selected to tap short-term visual and auditory memory, as well as verbal retrieval functions. These tasks included Sentence Repetition Test from the Detroit Test of Learning Aptitude, Digit Span from the age-appropriate Wechlser Intelligence Scale, Controlled Oral Word Association (FAS), and the Benton Visual Retention Test.

The Cognitive Domain was included to provide an overall appraisal of the individual's level of intellectual functioning. It was comprised of the Verbal IQ, Performance IQ, and Full Scale IQ from the age-appropriate Wechsler Scale.

Although these procedures were conceptually organized, each domain was subjected to data reduction strategies designed to determine whether the specified measures were sufficiently correlated to be summed meaningfully within each a priori domain. All scores were transformed into z-scores (ie., mean = 0, SD = 1). Table 1 shows the final composition of each domain of neuropsychological functioning that resulted when a principal components analysis, followed by a varimax rotation, was applied to the a priori hypothesized domains described above. Domain scores were computed as the mean of tests with loadings of 0.40 or greater in these analyses. Each domain summarized the information in the selected instruments well, with the proportion on variance accounted for ranging from 53% to 80%. Domain scores were computed as the average z-score from the specific tests incorporated into each domain.

Data Analyses. Two sets of analyses were conducted. The first evaluated whether the HIV-seropositve males performed significantly less well on the neuropsychologic assessment than did the HIV-seronegative group. The second set of analyses examined the relationship between neuropsychologic functioning and HIV-related illness, especially immune system compromise within the HIV+ group.

The first phase of analyses involved three sets of group comparisons. The first phase compared HIV+ and HIV- group mean domain scores using analyses of covariance, with maternal education and hemophilia severity included as potentially confounding covariates. These covariates were included because the HIV+ subjects were more likely to have mothers who averaged slightly less education and to have severe hemophilia than the HIV- group. When significant group mean differences on domain scores were detected, subsequent group comparisons of the individual measures comprising that domain score were made.

The second phase of data analysis evaluated whether either CD4 count or HIV-related illness classification was systematically related to neuropsychologic functioning for the 25 HIV- infected subjects. Each individual was placed into one of three categories on the basis of CD4 count: <200, 200 to 500, and> 500 cells/mm3. The CDC classification of symptomatic or asymptomatic disease was independently examined.

Results. Despite the use of three different strategies to address the question of group difference, these analyses revealed no neuropsychologic domains in which the

Table 1
Principal components analysis of neuropsychologic measures

Domain Test	Loading component 1	Loading component 2
Fine-Motor		
G Pegboard (domain)	-0.86	
G Pegboard (nondomain)	-0.88	
Trail Making A	-0.75	
Trail Making B		-0.60
Manual Finger Tapping (dominant)		0.87
Manual Finger Tapping (nondomain)		0.84
VMI		0.56
% Total Variance (66%)	33%	33%
Attention		
GDS (total correct)	0.82	
GDS (total commission)	-0.77	
GFW Selective Attention	0.66	
Wechsler Freedom From Distractibility*	0.64	
% Total Variance	53%	
Visual Processing		
Judgment Line Orientation	0.87	
Wechsler Perceptual Organization*	0.81	
Benton Visual Retention	0.77	
VMI test	0.70	
% Total Variance	62%	
Memory		
Wechsler Digit Span*	0.79	
Detroit Sentence Imitation	-0.84	
F-A-S Word Fluency	0.65	
Benton Visual Retention		0.88
% Total Variance (71%)	45%	26%
Language		
PPVT-R	0.92	
Wechsler Verbal Comprehension*	0.90	
GFW Auditory Discrimination	0.60	
% Total Variance	67%	
Cognition		
Wechsler Full-Scale IQ*	0.99	
Wechsler Verbal IQ*	0.91	
Wechsler Performance IQ*	0.91	
% Total Variance	80%	

GDS, Gordon Diagnostic System; PPVT, Peabody Picture Vocabulary Test - Revised; VMI, Developmental Test of Visual-Motor Integration.
*Wechsler = WISC-R or WAIS-R, depending on age of subject.
Taken from Whitt et al. (1993). With permission.

Table 2
Neuropsychologic domain scores for HIV+ and HIV- groups:
Summary scores from three analyses

	Group means*		%Pathognomic signs†		% Intraindividual scatter‡	
Domain	HIV+ (n=25)	HIV- (n=33)	HIV+ (n=25)	HIV- (n=33)	HIV+ (n=25)	HIV- (n=33)
Fine-Motor						
Motor 1	0.06±0.81	-0.33±1.03	0	9	8	27
Motor 2	-0.46±0.96	-0.62±0.91	8	9	20	42
Attention	-0.43±0.93	-0.36±0.70	13	0	25	24
Visual Processing	-0.55±0.97	-0.54±0.92	4	3	8	21
Memory						
Memory 1	0.08±0.67	-0.06±0.80	0	0	16	9
Memory 2	-0.27±0.91	0.22±1.03	0	0	17	7
Language	-0.19±1.03	0.08±0.94	0	0	0	9
Cognition	-0.27±1.03	-0.04±0.95	0	3	0	0

*Values are expressed as mean + SD.
†Proportion scoring more than 2 SD below age norms.
‡Proportion with z scores more than 1 SD below Full-Scale IQ z score.
Taken from Whitt et al. (1993). With permission.

HIV+ group performed significantly less well than HIV- subjects. The first strategy compared the group means of the two groups. After controlling for maternal education and hemophilia severity, no evidence of any group differences was noted. As can be seen in Table 2, group comparisons of the six neuropsychologic domains revealed no tendency for the HIV+ group to perform more poorly than the HIV- group.

The possibility that analyzing summary domain scores rather than specific scores from the selected instruments may have masked relevant HIV group differences was explored in descriptive post hoc analyses. First, each test score was examined for HIV group differences, with maternal education and hemophilia illness severity included as covariates. Of the 22 tests, four indicated marginal group differences, but the HIV+ group outperformed the HIV- group on each of these measures. Second, inclusion of hemophilia severity as a covariate produced conservative group comparisons because all HIV+ males had severe hemophilia. Thus, another set of post hoc analyses was performed to determine whether the lack of group differences was related to inclusion of the hemophilia severity variable. No group differences were observed in post hoc analyses either when hemophilia severity was omitted or when the HIV+ males with severe hemophilia were compared.

A second method of group analysis, a pathognomonic signs approach, utilized blind inspection of each individual's protocol for significant deficits (ie., more than two standard deviations below the test average) within the domains of functioning relative to age norms. This approach sought to discover whether there might be a smaller number of individuals who had significant difficulties in one or more areas of performance, but whose cumulative impact on a group mean domain score was insufficient to allow detection. When an arbitrary standard of a > 12% frequency of individuals demonstrating deficits within the sample was used there were higher frequencies of deficit relative to age-norm expectations for performance on the Motor Domain (VMI, Trails B), Attention Domain (Gordon Diagnostic System Total Correct and Total Commissions, GFW Selective Auditory Attention), Visual Processing Domain (Judgment of Line Orientation), and Language Domain (GFW Auditory Discrimination), by the group of HIV-Infected group; however, equally frequent deficits were found for each of these areas of neuropsychologic functioning within the control group of HIV-seronegative individuals with hemophilia.

The third group comparison strategy, an inspection of intraindividual scatter of abilities, compared each test score to each individual's level of intellectual functioning as determined by Wechsler Full Scale IQ. This strategy would permit the identification of areas of lower relative functioning (i.e., more than one standard deviation below FSIQ) that might not become apparent in age-based comparisons - thus detecting, for example, a very bright individual who had a relative deficit manifested by low average memory functioning. As with the age-norm-based comparisons, this strategy identified a similar set of significant relative deficits within the HIV+ group. Once again, the frequency of these deficits within each area of functioning did not differentiate the HIV+ group from the HIV- group; that is, although there were indications that some HIV-infected individuals had significantly lower motor, attention, and visual processing abilities than expected based on their own level of intellectual functioning, these problems occurred just as frequently in the HIV-control group.

Two analyses examined the relationship between neuropsychologic functioning and HIV-related illness. First, the HIV+ subjects' neuropsychologic domain scores were contrasted between groups defined by CD4 count categorization as defined

Table 3
Neuropsychologic domain scores for HIV+ subjects by CD4 category

Domain	Score by CD4 count			
	<200 cells/mm³ (n=6)	200-500 cells/mm³ (n=10)	>500 cells/mm³ (n=9)	ρ
Fine-Motor				
Motor 1	0.36±0.68	0.08±0.79	0.02±0.95	0.59
Motor 2	-0.55±1.13	-0.66±1.04	-0.16±0.75	0.53
Attention	0.03±0.85	0.64±1.10	-0.44±0.88	0.43
Visual Processing	-0.66±1.27	-0.68±0.92	-0.34±0.90	0.73
Memory				
Memory 1	0.91±1.23	0.08±0.59	0.00±0.39	0.87
Memory 2	-0.15±0.59	-0.49±0.87	-0.10±1.12	0.63
Language	-0.38±1.10	-0.42±0.88	0.18±1.17	0.43
Cognition	-0.48±1.32	-0.28±0.99	-0.15±1.10	0.86

Values (except ρ values) are expressed as mean ± SD.
Taken from Whitt et al. (1993). With permission.

earlier. As can be seen in Table 3, no significant relationship was detected in this sample. When individual tests were examined descriptively, only one of the 22 instruments showed the hypothesized relationship. Individuals with a CD4 count of less than 200 cell/mm3 had lower VMI scores (mean = 2.00, SD = 1.11) than did either individuals with CD4 counts of 200 to 500 cells/mm3 (mean = -1.27, SD = 1.23) or those with a CD4 count of more than 500 cells/mm3 (mean = -0.52, SD = 1.07).

Second, neuropsychologic functioning was examined in accordance with Centers for Disease Control (CDC) AIDS-stage classification. Only 2 of the 25 HIV+ individuals had symptomatic disease at their initial assessment. No domain or individual measure showed a significant difference as a function of CDC AIDS-stage classification.

Follow-up Studies. As part of the longitudinal investigation conducted by Whitt *et al.* (1993), these subjects have been tracked over the course of four years with respect to their neuropsychologic functioning. At the two-year follow-up point, using a similar set of data analysis strategies, the two groups continued to be indistinguishable in terms of their neuropsychological functioning (Hooper, Whitt, Tennison *et al.,* 1993a). Further, utilizing growth curve technology to track change over time, the two groups did not differ in terms of their rate or patter of change. Most recently, initial data analyses of domain scores for the entire data set over the four years of the project revealed similar findings (Hooper, Whitt & Burchinal 1995). That is, the HIV+ group did not differ in any of the neuropsychological domain scores, nor did they manifest any significant differences in terms of their rates and patterns of change over time.

Other Studies. While the findings noted above seem to go against earlier findings of HIV individuals showing cognitive deterioration (e.g., Aylward *et al.,* 1992; Levenson *et al.,* 1992; Novello *et al.,* 1989; Stover *et al.,* 1990), they are consistent with more contemporary, well-controlled studies examining individuals with hemophilia. For example, initial results from the Hemophilia Growth and Development Study (Hilgartner, Donfield, Willoughby *et al.,* 1993) revealed that their HIV+ subjects were relatively free of HIV- related neuropsychological impairment at baseline and that observed differences from a general population reflected effects of hemophilia as a chronic illness (Loveland, Stehbens, Contant *et al.,* 1994).

In contrast, Sirois and Hill (1993) reported on a small number of subjects from the Hemophilia Growth and Development Study study (n = 11) in which they found that HIV+ children infected during their preschool years performed more poorly on measures of perceptually-related abilities, and demonstrated more deficient retest effects on tasks requiring visual-motor coordination and perceptual organization than those infected during their middle childhood. A higher rate of neurological problems also was exhibited for the younger infected group. Although representative of case study methodology, these findings do suggest that age of infection may be an important variable in examining the neuropsychological functioning of this population.

Psychosocial:

Given the reported concerns for neurological and neuropsychological impairment in individuals who are HIV seropositive, it would seem likely that these children and adolescents also would be prone to social and behavioral difficulties. These problems might occur directly from HIV infection of the central nervous system and/or from the secondary effects of having to cope with a life-threatening illness (Belfner, Krener & Miller, 1988). Some data are emerging with respect to HIV- seropositive children and adolescents showing attentional difficulties (Kairam, Kugler, Zawadski *et al.*, 1991); however, most studies have concentrated on causes and treatment. Consequently, there are relatively few data on behavioral adaptation in HIV-seropositive children and adolescents.

Symptoms of emotional distress have been reported in HIV-seropositive adults, and have included mood elevation and irritability, blunted and depressed affect, anxiety, apathy, social withdrawal, excessive alcohol and drug usage, and suicidal ideation (e.g., Catalan, Douzenis, Brener & Meadows, 1991). In fact, Chuang, Devins, Hunsley & Gill (1989) found that the degree of distress tended to vary with the staging of the disease. These investigators reported that adults with AIDS-related complex and asymptomatic HIV disease were significantly more distressed than those with AIDS, with both groups evidencing significant elevations of depression, mood disturbance, and trait anxiety. Approximately a decade ago Wolcott (1986) even suggested that these psychosocial difficulties actually were manifestations of significant neurological involvement; however, more recently, Wilkins, Robertson, Snyder *et al.* (1991) have generated data to suggest otherwise.

At present, few such behavioral data exist for children and adolescents, although some trends have begun to be noted. For example, the work of Papola *et al.* (1994) showed approximately 16% of their HIV+ sample to manifest emotional difficulties severe enough to warrant a psychiatric diagnosis, with most of these concerns reflecting affective symptoms and emerging around adolescence; however, as with other such studies, these findings are not necessarily generalizable to individuals with hemophilia – especially given evidence that individuals with hemophilia, as a group, tend to be relatively uninfluenced by psychosocial factors (Handford, Mayes, Bixler & Mattison, 1986; Logan, Maclean, Howie *et al.*, 1990; Mayes, Handford, Kowalski & Schaefer, 1988). Nonetheless, Agle, Gluck & Pierce (1987) investigated the psychological impact of the risk of AIDS via a survey of 116 individuals with hemophilia, aged 16 and older, 40 spouses/mates, and 94 parents. These investigators found that, as a group, the population of individuals with hemophilia was coping effectively with the AIDS risk. They noted, however, that parents indicated more distress than either individuals with hemophilia or their mates. In fact, they suggested that increased parental anxiety could lead to over-protective child-rearing practices.

Perhaps one of the first published studies to address the behavioral adaptation of HIV-seropositive children and adolescents was conducted by Hooper, Whitt, Tennison *et al.* (1993b). Using the longitudinal sample described in the Whitt *et al.* (1993) study, the HIV+ and HIV- hemophilia groups were compared on the Child

Behavior Checklist (CBCL; Achenbach & Edelbrock, 1983). The CBCL is a parent rating measure designed to assess social competency and behavioural problems in children and adolescents. It is one of the most widely used measures of behavioural adjustment and has been used successfully with children and adolescents with chronic illness (Eiser, 1990).

The Social Competence Scale of the CBCL taps the parents' perceptions of their children's social involvement, the number and quality of social activities, and school performance. A Total Social Competency score also is generated. Similarly, the Behavior Problem or clinical scales provide summary scores for clusters of internalizing and externalizing behaviours, along with a Total Behavior Problem score. The Behavior Problem scales are subdivided into specific clinical scales and, for the purposes of this study include Uncommunicative, Obsessive-Compulsive, Somatic Complaints, Hyperactive, Aggressive, and Delinquent. These data were collected during the subject's inpatient admission for the longitudinal study. In addition to examining the group means on the social competency and clinical summary indices, the number of primary clinical scales with T-scores of 70 or higher for each individual was recorded and compared across the two groups. The groups also were compared in accordance with the three CD4 groups described above. Most of the CBCL's were completed by biological mothers (75%), with about one-quarter of the sample having CBCL's completed by fathers or other guardians.

Comparison of the HIV- seropositve and seronegative groups using analysis of covariance, with maternal education and severity of hemophilia as covariates, revealed no significant differences in parental ratings of social competencies. Similarly, no differences were noted between the groups on the clinical scales of the CBCL. The groups did not differ on the summary clinical indices, nor was there any significant differences on any of the specific clinical scales. There was no significant difference between the groups on the number of clinical scales that had scores of 70 or higher, and no significant trends were detected when the data were analyzed by CD4 group. In fact, the CBCL scores for both groups fell well within the normal range. These results can be seen in Table 4.

The results from the Hooper *et al.* (1993b) study were consistent with Sirois and Hill (1993) who found few documented social competency or behavioral problems on the CBCL in their small sample of HIV+ children and adolescents using the CBCL. Similarly, Hooper, Broder & Whitt (1997) were unable to document any major differences between their HIV+ hemophilia subjects and a sample of vertically-infected children and adolescents. Although the latter group was reported to have increased problems in the social domain, no significant differences were noted between the groups on the clinical scales. Similarly, using the Pediatric Behavior Scale (Lindgren & Koeppl, 1987), Loveland *et al.* (1994) found no significant differences between their HIV+ and HIV- groups in their baseline data from the Hemophilia Growth and Development Study.

Table 4
A Comparison of Human Immunodeficiency Virus (HIV) Seropositive (HIV+) and - Seronegative (HIV-) Children with Hemophilia on the Social Competence and Clinical Scales of the Child Behavior Checklist*

	Mean (+SD) Scores		
Scale	HIV+ (n=18)	HIV- (n=28)	*F*
Social Competence			
Activities	45.5±8.19	46.6±10.57	0.72
Social	42.4±9.74	46.0±5.72	0.62
School	47.1±8.28	45.2±9.34	0.61
Total	42.5±7.90	43.6±10.07	0.64
Clinical scales			
Uncommunicative	57.9±4.56	59.2±8.47	0.00
Obsessive-compulsive	59.2±8.55	60.8±7.68	0.46
Somatic complaints	61.0±7.04	61.4±7.22	0.19
Hyperactive	60.4±8.69	61.6±8.37	0.04
Aggressive	59.2±8.22	58.6±7.93	0.55
Delinquent	59.3±4.20	60.4±8.14	0.20
Internalized	53.8±11.5	56.5±11.04	0.32
Externalized	53.7±10.48	54.9±10.93	0.01
Total	54.5±11.13	57.0±11.52	0.04
No. of Clinical scales			
scoring ≥70	0.9+1.707	0.8+1.60	0.12

*All values are based on tests, with a mean (±SD) of 55+10. For the Social Competence scales, higher scores reflect more adaptive functioning. For the Clinical scales, lower scores reflect more adaptive functioning. The number of Clinical scales with scores of 70 or higher could range from 0 to 9. Taken from Hooper et al. (1993). With permission.

Summary

This section highlighted much of the available literature on the neuropsychological and psychosocial functioning of HIV+ adolescents with hemophilia. As can be seen from this review, relatively few data are available upon which to base clear conclusions as to the impact of HIV infection on the neuropsychological and social-emotional functioning of adolescents. The Whitt *et al.* (1993) study was described in some detail as it represented one of the first well-controlled studies to examine the neuropsychological functioning of HIV- seropositive children and adolescents with hemophilia, and it provided the foundation for the longitudinal tracking of this sample over a four year time span. In tandem with the emergent baseline results from the Hemophilia Growth and Development Study, findings to data would suggest that the impact of HIV-illness upon this population is not necessarily consistent with what has been reported to other groups of children and adolescents who are HIV- seropositive. More specifically, it would seem that a direct linkage between HIV- infection and neuropsychological or psychosocial functioning is not present in this population of individuals – at least those infected at a later age. Indeed, it would seem that the significant findings for the HIV+ group could be linked as much, if not more, to their chronic illness than to any primary impact of the HIV-infection on the central nervous system. The baseline data from the Whitt *et al.* (1993) and Loveland *et al.* (1994) studies, and the subsequent longitudinal findings by Hooper *et al.* (1993), Hooper *et al.* (1995), and Sirois & Hill (1993) all were consistent in this regard. These findings hold not only for the neuropsychological findings, but also for the psychosocial data. It would appear that there may be a plethora of other key issues at play when one considers the impact of HIV status on individuals with hemophilia.

ISSUES AND DIRECTIONS

Although the few published studies regarding the neuropsychological and social-emotional functioning of HIV-infected children and adolescents with hemophilia suggest that these individuals have incurred little or no direct impact from the HIV-related factors, there are a number of key issues that remain to be addressed at this time.

First, it is not an accident that there are not many studies examining this specific population of individuals. Although a major percentage of the severe hemophilia population was infected from their own treatment for hemophilia, actual numbers remain relatively small. In fact, the availability of samples such as those obtained in the Whitt *et al.* (1993) longitudinal study likely no longer exist due to the blood products screening and treatments and procedures that have been occurring for over a decade. These samples remain precious in terms of their ultimate outcome; hopefully, the continued study of these individuals will shed clues on their overall functioning as well as the ultimate impact of AIDS on the central nervous system. More specifically, with respect to the adolescent hemophilia population, there are few, if any, studies which have focused exclusively on an adolescent sample. This is because of the sampling problems which limit accrual of sufficient numbers to conduct appropriate data analyses.

Second, is the individual who is infected with HIV during early childhood different in terms of developmental attainment during adolescence than the individual infected during middle childhood? Are either of these individuals different than an individual who is infected during the adolescent years? On what parameters might they be different? It is argued that all of these cases could be discussed under the umbrella of adolescence, although the neuropsychological and psychosocial outcomes likely will be different for each of the different scenarios (e.g., age at infection, duration of illness, age at symptomatic onset of AIDS, etc.). Studies examining these issues need to be conducted.

For example, the time of infection may be crucial with respect to neurodevelopmental phenomena. In many respects, it is suspected that the impact of AIDS may not be unlike the impact that one might see from traumatic brain injury early in life (Levin *et al.*, 1984), wherein one's overall functioning has the potential to be compromised. Further, although the current studies did not document neurobehavioral or psychosocial changes in accordance with indices of disease severity (e.g., CD4 counts), recent evidence has suggested that specific behavioral change may be related more to the *rate* of change in CD4 count as opposed to the actual number of neurons destroyed. Although this has been suggested in the adult literature (Bornstein, Nasrallah, Para *et al.*, 1991), a parallel study has not been reported for children or adolescents.

Third, the methodological issues inherent in the study of this population are paramount. Even with a relatively fine-tuned neuropsychological examination, few significant differences have been noted between HIV+ and HIV- groups of children and adolescents with hemophilia. Nonetheless, had a control group of HIV-seronegative individuals with hemophilia not been employed in the studies by Whitt *et al.* (1993) and Loveland *et al.* (1994), a different set of conclusions might have been asserted. The importance of obtaining well-matched comparison groups cannot be overstated. Further, the use of growth curve technology also affords investigators the opportunity to examine longitudinal data sets for subtle changes over time that might otherwise be masked by use of more traditional change scores or other methods of analysis. Again, in the studies conducted to date with this population, the use of this statistical technology has not uncovered any significant differences between HIV+ and HIV- groups of individuals with hemophilia.

Fourth, issues pertinent to child/adolescent and family adaptation to chronic illness seem crucial to this population. As a group, adolescents with hemophilia have been reported to reflect a rather healthy social and emotional profile, and their level of intellectual functioning has been reported to be higher than average (Mayes *et al.*, 1988); however, this does not negate the fact that these individuals may not lead the "normal life" enjoyed by many of their peers. Their participation in contact sports is off-limits, and even their involvement in neighborhood games may be curtailed, thus limiting the number and types of social activities in which they might become engaged. Having HIV, or simply the chance that they might acquire AIDS, clearly adds additional burden to the stress of having a chronic illness such as hemophilia. For example, an important aspect of adolescent development is the cultivating of social, as well as intimate, relationships with the opposite gender. Not only is this normal adolescent goal hindered in the individual with hemophilia, as sharing this information may make it difficult to establish such relationships, but for the adolescent with hemophilia and HIV, developing such relationships can become even more problematic.

Although no differences were noted in behavioral competency at this point in time, observations of individual children and adolescents suggest the likelihood of affective and behavioral changes as progression of HIV symptomatology leads to the diagnosis of AIDS and alters the current therapeutic and family system routines. The numerous issues which confront these individuals and their families as AIDS symptomatology progresses (e.g., threat to life, emergent learning problems, disclosure of AIDS diagnosis to schools and other community agencies, social isolation or decreased peer involvement) may significantly jeopardize the "adaptive denial" which often characterizes the effective coping of children and adolescents with chronic illness and their families. Further, if compromised neurologic status does occur, it also may increase the risk that secondary social-emotional distress may become more extensive (Breslau & Marshall, 1985).

Fifth, it will be important to continue to examine the effects of pharmacological treatment upon the social-emotional and neuropsychological functioning in this population. Initial findings with such medications as Zidovudine (AZT) and Dideoxycytidine (ddC) suggest the potential for dramatic improvements in children's cognitive abilities (Pizzo, Butler, Balis *et al.*, 1990; Pizzo, Eddy, Falloon *et al.* 1988; Brouwers *et al.*, 1992), and it has been speculated that there will be a concomitant improvement in social and emotional status as well (Moss, Wolters, Eddy *et al.*, 1989). Hopefully, these medications alone or in combination with each other, or even in combination with other psychotropic medications (Walling & Pferrerbaum, 1990), will minimize the cognitive, social-emotional, and general adaptive difficulties apparent in this adolescent population. The development of new pharmocological agents undoubtedly will appear in the new future as well.

Sixth, in tandem with medical interventions, it will be important to address other aspects of the adolescent's life. For example, special education planning needs to be considered for this population. Although the actual intellectual and academic functioning of individuals with hemophilia may be higher than average, the impact of HIV-related issues may interfere with the demonstration of these competencies. Providing additional assistance to this group of adolescents, when needed, may preserve their academic self-esteem and enhance their quality of life.

Another example falls under the rubric of mental health care. Although the available data would suggest that the social and emotional impact of HIV-illness on adolescents with hemophilia appears minimal at present, especially if they incurred the infection at a later point in life, many of these individuals will struggle with the social-political issues that continue to be tied to the AIDS virus (e.g., discrimination), and these struggles undoubtedly will contribute ongoing stress to their lives. Further, social-emotional functioning may be mediated by family functioning and adaptation, as well as the various developmental challenges which face adolescents. For example, such positive outcomes may not be as evident in adolescents who became HIV- infected via vertical transmission, especially those who suffered the loss of a significant family member (e.g., a parent) to AIDS. Evaluation of these contextual and developmental components, measured in tandem with the direct impact of HIV-related disease on neurologic and immunologic functioning, will direct us toward effective strategies to support the continued behavioral competence of HIV-infected children and adolescents. Indeed, an entire issue of the *Journal of Adolescent Health* was devoted to increasing our understanding of these concerns (Kunins, Hein, Futterman, Tapley & Elliot, 1993).

Lastly, the avenue of prevention should continue to be explored. Education about HIV transmission and HIV- related issues continues to be important to the adolescent population. Indeed, Mason, Olson, Myers, Huszti and Kenning (1989) found in their survey of 132 patients with hemophilia and their families that most of the individuals wanted to know more information about the treatment of AIDS and how to cope with the stressors of AIDS. Although most of the patients reported that they had received adequate information about the transmission of the virus, many misconceptions were noted.

Although the findings by Mason *et al.* (1989) indicate the need for more education, there is a large body of evidence to suggest that information alone is not enough to produce the desired changes in decision making and behavioral practices (Brown, Nassau & Levy, 1990; Overby, Lo & Litt, 1989). Fisher and Fisher (1992) provided a model for the evolution of educational programs for the prevention of HIV infection in children and adolescents. They stated that any effective program for AIDS prevention should contain three major components. These include (1) information about AIDS transmission and prevention including addressing misconceptions that contribute to inappropriate fears of persons with AIDS; (2) motivational factors relevant to AIDS risk reduction such as perceived vulnerability, and (3) behavioral skills for engaging in practices associated with risk reduction. Siegel (1993) also noted that any such program should take into consideration the individual's conceptual understanding of AIDS and HIV-related issues (e.g., transmission). In this manner, it is hoped that prevention programs will continue to exert a positive influence on the attitudes, decision-making, and behavioral practices of adolescents with hemophilia.

CONCLUSIONS

This chapter has provided an overview of the literature on adolescents with hemophilia and HIV. It has highlighted the domains of neuropsychologic and social-emotional functioning with key studies being presented. Particular emphasis was placed on one logitudinal study which followed children and adolescents over a four year time frame. A number of key issues were discussed, including methodological and clinically relevant issues, with a particular eye toward future directions. It is hoped that this overview has opened a clearer path on which to continue our clinical and research efforts on adolescents with hemophilia and HIV/AIDS.

ACKNOWLEDGEMENTS

This chapter was supported by grants PO1 NS26680 from the National Institute of Neurological Disorders and Stroke; RR00046 from the University of North Carolina General Clinical Research Center; 90DD0207 from the Administration on Developmental Disabilities; and MCJ-379154-02-0 from the Maternal and Child Health Bureau.

REFERENCES

Achenbach, T. & Edelbrock, C. (1983) *Manual for the child Behavior Checklist and Revised Child Behavior Profile.* Burlington, VT: University of Vermont.

Agle, D., Gluck, H. & Pierce, G.F. (1987) The risk of AIDS: Psychologic impact on the hemophiliac population. *General Hospital Psychiatry.* **9**: 11-17.

Aylward, E. H., Butz, A.M., Hutton, N., Joyner, M. L., & Vogelhut, J. W. (1992) Cognitive and motor development in infants at risk for human immunodeficiency virus. *American*

Journal of Diseases of Children. **146**: 218-222.

Belfer, M. L., Krener, P. K. & Miller, F. B. (1988) AIDS in children and adolescents. *Journal of the American Academy of Child and Adolescent Psychiatry.* **27**: 147-151.

Bornstein, R. A., Nasrallah, H.A., Para, M.E. *et al.* (1991) Rate of CD4 decline and neuropsychological performance in HIV infection. *Archives of Neurology.* **48**: 704-707.

Breslau, N. & Marshall, I. A. (1985) Psychological disturbance in children with physical disabilities: Continuity and change in a 5-year follow-up. *Journal of Abnormal Child Psychology.* **13**: 199-216.

Brouwers, P., Moss, H., Wolters, P. *et al.* (July, 1992) *Neurobehavioral correlations in symptomatic pediatric HIV disease.* Paper presented at the Fourth International Neuroscience of HIV infection Conference, Amsterdam, The Netherlands.

Brouwers, P., van der Vlugt, H., Moss, H., Wolters, P. & Pizzo, P. (1995) White matter changes on CT brain scan are associated with neurobehavioral dysfunction in children with symptomatic HIV disease. *Child Neuropsychology.* **1**.

Brown, L. K., Nassau, J. H., & Levy, H. (1990) "What upsets me about AIDS is"...: A survey of children and adolescents. *AIDS Education and Prevention.* **2**: 296-304.

Catalan, J., Douzenis, A., Brener, N. & Meadows, J. (1991, June) *Psychiatric disorder in HIV disease: Description of 200 referrals to a liaison psychiatry service.* Paper presented at the Neuroscience of HIV Infection Satellite Conference, Padua, Italy.

Chuang, H. T., Devins, G. M., Hunsley, J. & Gill, M.J. (1989) Psychosocial distress and well-being among gay and bisexual men with human immunodeficiency virus infection. *American Journal of Psychiatry.* **146**: 876-880.

Eiser, C. (1990) Psychological effects of chronic disease. *Journal of Child Psychology, Psychiatry, and Allied Disciplines.* **31**: 85-98.

Fisher, J. D. & Fisher, W. A. (1992) Changing AIDS-risk behavior. *Psychological Bulletin,* **111**: 455-474.

Handford, H. A., Mayes, S. D., Bixler, E. O. & Mattison, R. E. (1986) Personality traits of hemophiliac boys. *Developmental and Behavioral Pediatrics,* 7: 224-229.

Hilgartner, M. W., Donfield, S. M., Willoughby, A. *et al.* (1993) Hemophilia growth and development study. Design, methods, and entry data. *The American journal of Pediatric Hematology/Oncology,* **15**: 208-218.

Hooper, S. R., Broder, H. L. & Whitt, J. K. (1997) *Behavioral ratings of HIV-seropositive children and adolescents.* Manuscript in submission.

Hooper, S. R., Whitt, J. K. & Burchinal, M. (1995, March) *Neuropsychological functioning in HIV-infected children and adolescent with hemophilia: A four-year longitudinal study.* Paper presented at the Biennial General Conference of the Society for Research and Children Development, Indianapolis, Indiana.

Hooper, S. R., Whitt, J. K., Tennison, M. B. *et al.* (1993a, April) *HIV-infected children with hemophilia: One and two year follow-up neuropsychological functioning.* Paper presented at the Biennial General Conference of the Society for Research and Child Development, New Orleans, Louisiana.

Hooper, S.R., Whitt, J. K., Tennison, M. *et al.* (1993b) Behavioral adaptation to human immunodeficiency virus-seropositive status in children and adolescents with hemophilia. *American Journal of Diseases of Children,* **147**: 541-545.

Jason, J., Stehr-Green, J., Holman, R., Evatt, B. & the Collaborative Study Group (1988) Human immunodeficiency virus infection in hemophiliac children. *Pediatrics,* **82**: 565-570.

Kairam, R., Kugler, S., Zawadski, R. *et al.* (1991, June) *Range of neurological and psychological dysfunction in pediatric HIV infection.* Paper presented at the Neuroscience of HIV Infection Satellite Conference, Padua, Italy.

Kunins, H., Hein, K., Futterman, D. *et al.* (1993) Guide to adolescent HIV/AIDS program development. *Journal of Adolescent Health,* **14** (Special Issue).

Levenson, R. L., Mellins, C. A., Zawadzki, R. *et al.* (1992) Cognitive assessment of human immunodeficiency virus-exposed children. *American Journal of Diseases of Children,* **146**: 1479-1483.

Lindgren S. & Koeppl, G. K. (1987) Assessing child behavior problems in a medical setting: Development of the Pediatric Behavior Scale. In R. Prinz (Ed.), *Advances in behavioral assessment of children and families* (Vol. 3, pp. 57-90). Greenwich, CT: JAI.

Logan, F. A., Maclean, A., Howie, C.A. *et al.* (1990) Psychological disturbance in children with hemophilia. *British Medical Journal,* **301**: 1253-1256.

Loveland, K. A., Stehbens, J., Contant, C. *et al.* (1994) Hemophilia growth and development study: Baseline neurodevelopmental findings. *Journal of Pediatric Psychology,* **19**: 223-239.

Mason, P. J., Olson, R.A., Myers, J. G., Hustzi, H.C. & Kenning, M. (1989) AIDS and hemophilia: Implications for interventions with families. *Journal and Pediatric Psychology,* **14**: 341-355.

Mayes, S. D., Handford, H.A., Kowalski, C. & Schaefer, J. H. (1988) Parent attitudes and child personality traits in hemophilia: A six-year longitudinal study. *International Journal of Psychiatry and Medicine,* **18**: 339-355.

Moss, H., Wolters, P., Eddy, J. *et al.* (1989) The effects of encephalopathy and AZT treatment on the social and emotional behavior in pediatric AIDS. *V International Conference on AIDS: Abstracts,* **5**: 328.

Novello, A. C., Wise, P. H., Willoughby, A. & Pizzo, P. A. (1989) Final report of the United States Department of Health and Human Services Secretary's Work Group on pediatric human immunodeficiency virus infection and disease: content and implication. *Pediatrics,* **84**: 547-555.

Overby, K. J., Lo, B. & Litt, I. F. (1989) Knowledge and concerns about acquired immunodeficiency syndrome and their relationship to behavior among adolescents with hemophilia. *Pediatrics,* **83**: 204-210.

Papola, P., Alvarez, M. & Cohen, H. J. (1994) Developmental and service needs of school-age children with human immunodeficiency virus infection: A descriptive study. *Pediatrics,* **94**: 914-918.

Pizzo, P. A., Butler, K., Balis, F. *et al.* (1990) Dideoxycytidine alone and in an alternating schedule with zidovudine in children with symptomatic human immunodeficiency virus infection. *Journal of Pediatrics,* **117**: 799-808.

Pizzo, P. A., Eddy, J., Falloon, J. *et al.* (1988) Effect of continuous intravenous infusion of zidovudine (AZT) in children with symptomatic HIV Infection. *New England Journal of Medicine,* **319**: 889-896.

Scott G. B. (1988) Clinical manifestations of HIV infection in children. *Pediatric Annals,* **17**: 365-370.

Siegel, L. J. (1993) Editorial: Children's understanding of AIDS: Implications for preventive interventions. *Journal of Pediatric Psychology,* **18**: 173-176.

Sirois, P. A., & Hill, S. D. (1993) Developmental change associated with human immunodeficiency virus infection in school-age children with hemophilia. *Developmental Neuropsychology,* **9**: 177-197.

Stehr-Green, J. K., Holman, R. C., Jason, J. M. & Evatt, B. L. (1988) Hemophilia-associated AIDS in the United States, 1981 to September 1987. *American Journal of Public Health,* **78**: 439-442.

Stover, E. S., Pequegnat, W., Huffman, L. *et al.* (1990) CNS aspects of HIV-1 infection and AIDS in infants and children: A collaborative research. *Pediatrics AIDS and HIV Infection from Fetus to Adolescence*, **6**: 109-120.

Tennison, M.B., Messenheimer, J. A., Ehle, A. L. *et al.* (1989, September) *Clinical neurophysiologic assessment of children seropositive for HIV-1.* Paper presented at the American Electroencephalographic Society Annual Meeting, New Orleans, Louisiana.

Walling, V. R. & Pfefferbaum, B. (1990) The use of methylphenidate in a depressed adolescent with AIDS. *Journal of Developmental and Behavioral Pediatrics*, **11**: 195-197.

Whitt, J. K., Hooper, S. R., Tennison, M. B. *et al.*, (1993) Neuropsychologic functioning of human immunodeficiency virus-infected children with hemophilia. *Journal of Pediatrics*, **122**: 52-59.

Wilkins, J. W., Robertson, K. R., Snyder, C. R. *et al.* (1991) Implications of self-reported cognitive and motor dysfunction in an HIV+ inpatient population. *American Journal of Psychiatry*, **148**: 641-643.

Wolcott, D. L. (1986) Neuropsychiatric syndromes in AIDS and AIDS-related illnesses. In L. McKusick (Ed.), *What to do about AIDS: Physicians and mental health professionals discuss the issues* (pp. 32-44). Los Angeles: University of California Press.

11

Adaptation and Coping of HIV Infected Adolescents Living in France

ISABELLE FUNCK-BRENTANO, FLORENCE VEBER, MARIANNE DEBRE & STEPHANE BLANCHE

INTRODUCTION

By September 1996 the cumulative number of persons diagnosed with AIDS was 45,204 – 666 of these were children. France, Spain and Italy have become the three countries with the highest rate of HIV infected children in western Europe. According to international data on the natural history of HIV disease in children, 75% of the infected children are alive at the age of 6, the majority of whom are healthy with few biological and/or clinical signs of disease. During this time period, a slight morbidity is still reported. Some of these children were infected through contaminated blood transfusion or during treatment of haemophilia before the year 1985. Disease progression in these children is similar in many ways to the course of the disease in vertically infected children, although some uncertainties still remain. Nowadays most infection in children is through materno-foetal transmission and today, very few young adolescents would be expected to have been infected through sexual contact or intravenous drug use. This paper is based on an evaluation of experience with 50 adolescents among the 400 HIV infected children followed in Necker-Enfants Malades hospital, Paris, France. Most are still in the early stage of adolescence, i.e. 12 or 13 years old. By 1996 the oldest vertically infected children were over 16 years old and several children who had been contaminated through blood transfusion had already reached adulthood.

COGNITIVE DEVELOPMENT AND SCHOOL ACHIEVEMENT

Blanche *et al.* (1990) describes a bimodal expression of the disease which predicts that about 80% of the infected children develop a slowly progressive form of the disease. During this phase, which can last for several years, they remain asymptomatic or have reversible symptoms. All the surviving adolescents belong to this category of disease. The other 20% infected children developed a severe form of the disease with severe neurological symptoms, mental retardation and death before the age of 6. In the slowly progressive form, cognitive development appears to be within the normal ranges for most of the children and school performance is good in 2/3 of the elementary school-aged children (Tardieu *et al.*, 1995; Tardieu, in press; Funck-Brentano, 1996). However, selective visual-spatial impairment has been frequently observed, and eventual long term consequences on academic achievement should be studied. Early data had shown that 44% to 90% of the children were cognitively impaired (Diamond, 1989; Levenson *et al.*, 1992; Armstrong *et al.*, 1993; Mellins *et al.*, 1994; Cohen *et al.*, 1991; Colegrove Huntzinger, 1994; Papola *et al.*, 1994). However, these studies had numerous methodological problems which may account for the differences. They had mixed the two categories of children, which led to an increased number of children with developmental delay in the sample. Moreover prenatal drug exposure may have an impact on cognitive development. Such drug use factors may occur more frequently in the United States. Drug use is known to increase the risk of developmental delay for children complemented by other factors such as low birth weight and low socioeconomic status (Mellins *et al.*, 1994). In the French cohort of 50 adolescents cognitive development appears within normal ranges and the majority of adolescents are attending high school as appropriate. When visual-spatial impairment or a learning disability was diagnosed at elementary school age, the children were usually provided with a specialised programme. Several children have required such programmes and at four year follow up school performance is good. A small number had to be held back one year. Five of the adolescents with AIDS are attending school part-time, because they are too tired or because treatments are time consuming and not compatible with a standard timetable. Only a few adolescents have needed to repeat one or two years because of frequent illness resulting in poor school attendance. Currently, the oldest 16 year old girls are performing very well at their age appropriate level. A young adult, now aged 25, had decided to give up school when he turned 16 in order to enjoy life freely given that he was healthy. He devoted himself to social activism, relying on his parent for his financial needs.

In summary, from the French experience, it can be expected that a number of adolescents will attend high school and will graduate to university or occupational level after having proceeded with training of their choice. This is only when not affected by disease progression or intense treatment procedures.

Nutritional problems may necessitate support with either enteral or parenteral nutrition, using a nasogastric tube or a catheter connected to a feed-pump. Extension of home care programmes including training and involvement of the parents can sometimes help avoid hospitalization, which would be detrimental to family functioning and the child's mental health. Thus, when practical and psychological constraints allow, nutritional support has been shown to improve the quality of life of a number of children who become able to live a normal life, attending school and social activities on a regular basis (Goulet, in press; Funck-Brentano, in press). Longitudinal studies should extend experience and knowledge on the cognitive abilities and academic achievement of HIV infected adolescents as well as the quality of life of those who are undergoing home care programmes such as nutritional support.

Although encephalopathy does not usually occur after 3 years of age, 2 adolescents suffered from a progressive encephalopathy persisting until their death. They showed symptoms of rapid motor and mental deterioration similar to the early severe form of the disease in children, or to acquired dementia described in adults. It occurred after the onset of AIDS, invariably as a consequence of secondary lesions of the CNS due to opportunistic infections such as Cytomegalovirus or Papovavirus. A few adolescents have been described as having experience of vascular and ischemic lesions. Sometimes the occurrence of a sensorial deficit, such as visual loss, adds another disability with a poor prognosis. Six adolescents had occasional or persistent psychiatric disorders diagnosed as brief psychotic disorder with hallucinations and confusion sometimes associated with parkinsonian symptoms, acute psychosis with delirium and hallucinations which persisted in 1 child until death.

Psychiatric disorders sometimes precede neurologic symptoms such as bipolar depressive and manic disorders with conduct disorder without mental deterioration, anxiety and depressive disorders similar to adults (Tardieu (in press), Funck-Brentano (in press)). Clearly a prospective study to explore the origin and course of adolescent psychiatric disorders is desirable to address much uncertainty and ignorance which remains. Despite their relative rare occurrence, experience with adults would lead to hypotheses that psychiatric disorders in adolescents will increase over time as adolescents reach adulthood.

PSYCHOLOGICAL ADJUSTMENT AND EMOTIONAL NEEDS

Adolescence is often described as a time of major physical and mental change. The consequence may result in an extremely ambivalent position between aggressiveness and positive affective feelings. Some theories propose that this is a sign of an effective close dependency on the family. Many psychological explanations of adolescent psyche may be complicated by the presence of disease. When the physical condition in an adolescent deteriorates, they can be exposed to death anxieties. These traditionally would encourage closer proximity to the family for protection. Sick adolescents may need to integrate a new adult body image for the future, to accommodate a new relationship with their own future sexuality and with their environment. This may be challenging at a time when they are very reluctant to address these issues, given that they are exposed to physical changes produced by the disease, often accompanied by muscular weakness; functional limitations and feelings of frailty or insecurity. Such exposure may promote regressive tendencies. New opportunities may not be challenges but may be perceived as threatening. In this situation of major vulnerability, the quality of the relationships between the adolescents, their families, and health carers is crucial and will either elicit or impede the mental and cognitive structuring which has to be achieved by the adolescents to be able to cope with their disease and to resolve the adolescence crisis successfully.

Adjustment problems and psychiatric disorders in HIV infected children are influenced by 2 major factors such as:

- disease characteristics
- the quality of the family and caregiver's environment
- experience of adversive life events

These have been studied in a variety of settings (Papola, 1994; Cohen, 1994; Havens *et al.*, 1994; Bose *et al.*, 1994; Mellins & Enhardt, 1994; Wiener *et al.*, 1994). In general, children with psychiatric disorders have often experienced chaotic family circumstances with deprivation and neglect as reported by Cohen (1994) & Papola (1994). Experience with children and HIV is consistent with data which emphasises the role of negative background factors on psychological adjustment. Such background factors are common to many HIV infected children. Although it is known that children with chronic illness are at higher risk for psychiatric problems than are their healthy peers (Cadman *et al.*, 1987; Thompson *et al.*, 1989; Thompson, *et al.*, 1992), the rates of behavioural and psychiatric morbidity which are found in the HIV infected children and in their parents are often very high. The reasons for this are many including adverse background factors, HIV associated factors and the cumulative effects of adversity.

Child psychological disturbances can be related to the persistent traumatic impact of HIV on the parents. Looking at the various transmission routes, HIV infection brings with it a whole collection of anxieties and guilt feelings in parents which may be repeated and intensified as the disease progresses. HIV infection may affect several members of a family (often over two generations at the same time). These factors can predispose parents to long term reactive disorders. These disorders can result in disruptions of the parent-child relationship such as "mourning anticipation" or "affective anaesthesia" and rejection. In such cases parents are unresponsive to the needs of their children because they remain emotionally in shock and convinced that their child is soon going to die. Over-protective behaviour can also disturb child development as the child is growing in a negative atmosphere fraught with anxiety and vulnerability. In such circumstances parents may be neither able to reflect a positive self-image to their child nor make plans for his or her future. Therefore, early disruptions in parents or caregivers-child relationships can take place and persist in the long term as a consequence of HIV.

Thus, when children enter adolescence, many of them present specific personality characteristics such as inhibition, severe immaturity and unresolved dependency on the mother. Such dependency can be acutely oriented to the physical presence of the mother and exclude various attachments to other people. In these situations, socialization is often restricted. Such children make few friends and they do not enjoy going to school. These children also show depressive disturbances, anxiety, helplessness, attachment requests and difficulties in identification. Conflicts or interpersonal problems with family members are more sporadic. They occur mainly when a parent is also infected, especially when acceptance of their own medical condition is an issue. For example a father who denies his own infection or sickness can develop aggressive attitudes toward his infected child who reflects his own health status back to him. In return, the child rebels against the father by means of various behavioural disturbances. In some cases, children can complain of physical symptoms which are not fully explained by their HIV infected condition, and psychological factors are involved. In our experience these features and tendencies exist in at least half of the infected adolescents, and when they do, they are rather pervasive. They are unrelated to the transmission route and to the clinical status of the children, even though progression of the disease usually exacerbates the impaired parent-child interaction.

Finally, a few parents or caregivers reject their infected child, either because they cannot tolerate caring for a sick child or because they fear that the HIV infected child might infect their healthy children if he/she were to remain at home. In such cases, children receive care from foster families or medical institutions, while health professionals combine their efforts to maintain as a relationship as possible between the child and the family. In some of these fraught situations the children spontaneously request separation from their family. This is documented when children have experienced repeated neglect. In practice, once the withdrawal and alternative placement is accomplished, many children initially express feelings of relief. These solutions may be short term or problematic, as exposure to deprivation and rejection will almost certainly have left the child vulnerable. Separation problems may well persist for some time, even into adulthood.

Adverse life events experienced over several generations in the family can affect the child, who is exposed to the weight of past difficulties inherited from his or her family members. These include a number of experiences such as early neglect or maltreatment, disruptive family environment and multiple separations, drug use, medical antecedent other than HIV, economic and social problems, uprooting and social adjustment problems for migrant parents. In addition, for some parents, these problems are heightened by their medical condition, economic crisis factors and their immigrant status. These adverse family life events can be detrimental to the next generation of children who experience similar neglect and deprivation. This context of disruption and suffering can trigger feelings of insecurity, depression and anxiety for any child irrespective of their medical status. Some of them react with severe disorders in early infancy, such as pervasive developmental disorder and reactive attachment disorder. Once they received care from extended or foster families, or an institution, with emotional support, they may succeed in adjusting to their future demands. Therapeutic intervention may be required to allow their adjustment to improve sufficiently for them to continue with full social lives and school attendance. Support may not be a guaranteed cure, and many children may continue to exhibit vulnerability, with separation anxiety and behavioural problems.

Problems tend to be emphasized in the adolescence stage with the reappearance of conflicts, depressive affects, difficulties with identification process and reluctance to comply with independence and autonomy. In actual fact, when looking at the emotional life of children and adolescents, some are only suffering from detrimental environmental circumstances while others are affected by their medical condition, and yet others by a complex interaction of both factors.

Many HIV infected adolescents are confronted with occasional or recurrent subjective distress directly related to HIV. This includes a multitude of possible feelings such as those associated with low self-esteem, helplessness, injured self-image related to functional disabilities, worries about progression of the disease, death anxiety for themselves or their parents, problems with the constraints of various treatments and some invasive investigations, intolerance of hospital dependency, fear of re-experiencing physical pain which is still traumatic in their memory; unease following the manner in which they were informed about the disease, fear of threats and hostility from their social environment should their HIV status become known. Home care programs have improved the quality of life of children and their families but the underlying constraints relating to intensive treatment procedures can also be problematic for the family. Home programmes may need constant evaluation and readjustment.

The psychological state of children or adolescents reaching terminal stage is varied. Some are well adjusted while in other cases a sudden new event can render the situation unendurable, especially for those who are already very weak. In such circumstances, health carers should concentrate all their resources towards improving the comfort of the adolescent. Key elements of attention surround pain management, treatment of anxiety and/or depression, psychological support, physical care such as massage and relaxation and arrangements to facilitate the stable presence of the mother, or her substitute. It should be added that the parents' health status and the progression of their disease is crucial in child and adolescent psychological functioning. When a parent's life is ending, all family members are confronted with acutely stressful situations highlighting separation and loss anxieties. Ultimately death comes, to conclude this period of uncertainty. Family life can function again, with extended family members who are again available for the children. In our experience most bereaved adolescents lost their parents when they were younger, and many of them have been raised by their extended family for several years. This data is clearly monitored in the French prospective study conducted between 1986 and 1993 (Blanche *et al.*, 1996). With respect to HIV infection, the classical conception of family had to be put aside in order to embrace new kinds of family units, which were unusual in the context of chronic illness such as single families, extended family with grandparents, aunts and uncles or foster families.

Repeated deaths within the same family and disruptive family environments have often led to a frailty of ties and relationships in quite a number of families. Bereaved children cared for by grandparents can face generational differences with different approaches to child rearing or because grandparents are not sufficiently empowered to play the substitute role of the parents. Sometimes one parent is still alive but is totally unable to care for his/her children because of a disruptive lifestyle, drug use or physical disabilities related to HIV. Then the grandparents often take care both of the sick parent and the children, a situation which is uncomfortable for all family members. When parents in terminal stage are cared for by medical institutions, visits of their children are organized to maintain, at the least, a minimal relationship between them. But children and adolescents find it distressing to see a debilitated parent and they often prefer to stay away. One of them recently stated that he did not want to visit his mother anymore and that he did not wish to be told about her death when it happens. This boy had suffered for a long time from deep resentment against his mother, while his father who was very close to him had died several years ago. In such cases, it is helpful to offer the child and the dying parent an opportunity to communicate and share important feelings and thoughts. This can create a helpful basis from which the mourning processes can be initiated.

Several grandparents who had failed in raising their children have been surprisingly successful in caring for their grandchildren. Time and experience have shown them their past deficiencies and they have learned from a situation which gives them an opportunity to make up for the mistakes they felt they had made with their own children. They are challenged by a dramatic situation in which both children and grandchildren are infected, and there is probably strong pressure on them to play the role of a good parent in rescuing their grandchildren. Experience shows that they are usually successful in their attempt. Nevertheless, as the years pass, grandparents can easily begin to feel overwhelmed, because their childrearing time has passed. Indeed this involvement may begin to conflict with their personal needs as they grow older. They grow easily tired and start to complain and exaggerate small everyday problems. Such reactions should be monitored as signs that the task they have taken on is beginning to worry them, even though it had been initially welcome. When grandchildren start to misbehave, the revival of past conflicts between the grandparents and their children may elicit ambivalence towards their grandchildren, a situation which may lead to interpersonal conflicts. For the children, many of whom are still young, they may have replacement parents, but can feel a loss of grandparents. They may also worry about their grandparents health and how much longer they might have to live. Therefore, provision of support and counselling is especially necessary in order for the grandparents to maintain the ability, motivation and confidence to cope with their grandchildren.

A number of questions are raised about the future of orphaned children who are cared for by the extended family: long term consequences of the losses of their parents and siblings, confusion between parental and grandparental images, the quality of identification images supported by grandparents alone, the impact of HIV infection on the adolescent's ability to consider the future including sexual behaviour and to take on adult responsibilities.

Many of the adolescents grow more slowly as a result of HIV associated with nutritional problems. As a result, some have failed to thrive, experience delayed puberty and are often immature. Few receive early sex education to prevent the spread of the disease. Nevertheless some girls are already pubescent and they can be considered as being at risk of transmission of the virus if they were to become sexually active. Then the responsibility to protect them from infection and to protect their partners becomes an important issue. Prevention of sexual transmissions raises major questions about perceptions of the disease from the adolescent's perspective and on the ways their infection or disease is explained to them.

DISCLOSURE AND ADOLESCENT'S PERCEPTION OF THE DISEASE

In most care centers, it is generally agreed that the right to disclose to or conceal from a child his/her HIV diagnosis belongs to the child's caregiver. In such cases, information to the children about the illness is always provided either by the parents or by the physician. This should be preceded by discussion of this issue with the parents in agreements on the contents of disclosure.

Although it is assumed that adolescents are more mature than children, experience shows that many parents still view the disclosure issue from the same perspective as for younger children. Thus, HIV infection still confronts health professionals with a conflict between the children's need and right to receive information about their health status, and the parent's right and duty to protect their children from threatening information and from discriminatory reactions from society.

It is generally agreed that basic and understandable information should be provided at any age to sick children so that medical care can make sense to them. This facilitates their participation in, and acceptance of, the investigations and treatment procedures. Opinion is often unclear on the extent of disclosure – including AIDS diagnosis – before the adolescent stage. Many health professionals believe that telling children of their HIV infection or AIDS diagnosis gives them little benefit and could bring them unnecessary difficulty. Nowadays HIV infection is linked in the mind of every child to the concept of death, so telling children who are HIV infected, but clinically well, may generate inappropriate early death anxieties. One has to keep in mind that only children with enough maturity are able to distinguish the stage of infection from the disease stage, a difference which is even not easily understood in adults. Moreover, disclosure of HIV/AIDS diagnosis requires that children are mature enough to understand concepts of secrecy and stigma. If children do not understand the reasons for this recommendation, they might experience distress with feelings of shame, guilt or isolation leading to a worse situation than before they learnt of their infection.

Lies or nondisclosure creates anxiety in the children and lead to noncompliant attitudes, even when they seem to have tacitly absorbed and followed the family code of silence. Similarly attitudes of denial on the part of the parents or the physician could be experienced by the children as sharing the helplessness of their carers, and at worse as a kind of abandonment, in this way a greater burden would be added to their distress. During the past decade, health professionals have become more and more convinced that using partial disclosure with HIV infected preschoolers and elementary school-aged children is the most appropriate way to talk to them about their infection/disease (Funck-Brentano, 1996; Lipson, 1994; Hardy *et al.*, 1994). Partial disclosure includes a description of symptoms and treatments and an understanding of the virus and the immunodificiency mechanism. Children are given explanations such as being told that they are lacking in white cells or immune defences and this is the reason why they cannot fight microbes or viruses efficiently. Pills or medicines, injections of antibiotics or veinoglobulines are required to help them fight against these enemies and to reinforce their internal system of defense. This pattern of disclosure is consistent with the corresponding stage of children's understanding of illness causality as concrete logical explanations according to the Piagetian model (Perrin, *et al.*, 1991; Bibace & Walsh, 1980; Brewster, 1982; Walsh & Bibace, 1991; Springer, 1994). A recent investigation conducted in one of the major hospitals in France caring for HIV infected children has shown that 70% of the children under 12 years of age had partial knowledge of their infection/disease. This demonstrates an increased propensity of pediatricians and parents to use partial disclosure. Currently, quite a number of adolescents still show this pattern of disclosure, even though they have reached a formal-logical level of understanding. A number of reasons can explain this phenomenon. Parents are still very reluctant to reveal to a child his or her HIV status because it would bring up death anxieties and lead to questions about transmission route, an issue which is greatly feared by HIV infected parents as well as by parents of transfusion infected children. In some cases they feel persecuted, with acute guilt related to their failure to protect their child from the transmission of the virus, even though they had no knowledge of the danger at that time. As a result they cannot bear to acknowledge their failure by talking about the cause of infection with their children. These feelings are particularly overwhelming in mothers of haemophiliac children as their initial experience of guilt, relating to their responsibility in the transmission of haemophilia, was reinforced once again by a fatal medical procedure they had initially requested and signed for. When the parents are infected, disclosure would suggest to the children that their parent might die, abandoning them too early, another argument for the parents to defend an attitude of nondisclosure. Finally, revealing how the parents became infected risks disclosing past life events or behaviour that they may wish to keep secret. Such unspoken reasons support parental disclosure resistance. Currently, in our experience, the AIDS diagnosis has been disclosed to 80% of children 13 years old and over and to 40% of children between 10 and 13 years old. Very few children know their diagnosis before they are 10 years old.

Our experience (Funck-Brentano, 1994) as well as literature (Lipson, 1993; Lipson, 1994; Bibace & Walsh, 1980; Brewster, 1982; Walsh & Bibace, 1991) shows that children under 12 years of age have little concern about their precise diagnosis. Rather, they worry about their symptoms with unpredictable concerns regarding causes and treatment procedures. While parents and health professionals either communicate by way of imagery or adopt a more scientific style, according to the child's age and maturity, in some cases usual terminology can bring up unexpected images which have a severe impact on children. For instance, a girl who had been told that microbes were responsible for her infection responded with unexpected anxiety to the word "microbe". In fact it turned out that she hated this word because she was nicknamed "Microbe" at school by her peers because she was small. Two children whose parents had died were very susceptible to separation experiences and they suffered from sleep disorders. When the purpose of the antiviral treatment was explained with reference to the idea "make the virus sleep", anxiety and distress emerged because they associated the word "sleep" with images of "separation" or "death". A 12 year old girl expected that the virus would leave her one day thanks to the blood extractions she was going through once a month, but she was scared that consequently all her blood would finally be removed from her body. Those anecdotes demonstrate that both children and adolescents can have unpredictable fantasies and worries triggered by very simple and common words. Consequently priority needs to be given to these concerns and inquiries which have to be discussed with the children prior to the diagnosis issue which is often not the children's main concern. Often opportunistic infections, symptoms or specific affections are perceived by the children as diagnosis of their disease. Actually children's and adolescents' images and fantasies about their body functioning and sickness are unique and innumerable. Thus following the individual path of questions and fantasies should be the basis of further information provision.

When parents are healthy, very few children and adolescents are aware of their parent's infection/disease and are often not aware of any link in their medical status. In some families, when parents are symptomatic, their children are partially aware of their parent's infection and several of them have noticed similarities between their common symptoms or treatments. Although they obviously receive clues which would lead to a realisation that the two diseases are identical, nevertheless most of the children avoid pursuing the analogy. It is plausible that children might have tacitly considered as dangerous for themselves and unbearable for their parents to think over similarities in symptoms and treatments. The tendency to minimize or deny the sickness of their parents can be observed in several children and can be interpreted as an attempt to protect themselves against awareness of their parent's weakness or the fear of their parent's death. Several children have shown fairly accurate understanding of the maternal transmission via drawings and comments without anything having been stated about it from their environment. A few children have been told that indeed they had the same sickness and its relation to maternal transmission.

Those children whose parents are in the terminal stage or have already died have been told about their parent's disease, and their own, in various ways. The death of a parent arouses many questions in children's minds among which are queries about the similarity of their diseases, the maternal transmission route and fear and anticipation of their own death. These thoughts and questions are either shared with the caregivers or discussed when children and caregivers are using problem solving strategies to cope with the problem (Brown, 1995). For some adolescents, intellectualizing the situation by naming the disease helps them to control their anxieties, while some of them may disguise conscious affects. For others, repression of affects and traumatic memories results in not recognizing or expressing relevant affects. In such cases, enactment of internal conflicts may occur, and without realizing it, the child or adolescent may continually reenact the original problem with people who are significant in his or her current life. This may perpetuate a continual state of frustration and interpersonal conflict. Actually more and more children become aware of the severity of their physical condition by understanding the link between the disease or death of a parent and their own infection. This tendency should increase as the number of dying parents rises over the coming years. Thus progressive disclosure should lead to full disclosure including Aids diagnosis as adolescents realize the nature of their disease and the physical and emotional experiences related to it. Naming the disease can be helpful in some cases, or at some times. At other periods the same child or adolescent may choose to use strategies such as wishful thinking, denial, or cleavage by projecting his or her sick body-parts on to the outside. Defense mechanisms which emerge for the child may serve a self-protective function by shielding the child and adolescent from the experience of fearful affects as their body suffers from successive detrimental changes.

Irrespective of physical disabilities, impairments or level of functioning, they have to cope with the infection or disease in order to develop their personality. Regular reliance on a physician and treatments may make the adolescents feel different from others and, simultaneously idealize the physician and health carers who have become indispensable to them. Adolescents may respond by creating a strong involvement with carers, by playing down the constraints which disturb, by pretending they are not interested in the information they are provided with about their disease, or by giving the impression that they don't know its name or the issues surrounding it. These strategies may help them avoid having to acknowledge the reality of their infection. Similarly they may use treatment sessions to create difficulties for the health carers. For some adolescents these various responses are the only means they have at their disposal to create a small space of personal freedom, control, expression, to deny their sickness and defy their health carers.

When they reach terminal stage, disclosure of diagnosis may be rather inadequate and intrusive at a time when the adolescent's needs are mainly centred on primary care, security and elective close relationships with the family. Feeling that life is ending, adolescents may stop the linking process of mental imagery about the disease, and completely avoid thinking about it. This defense mechanism shields them from an unbearable level of anxiety. It is not common to observe cases where mental processes are paralysed and compliance with the unspoken social attitudes operates as a fundamental protective mechanism.

Multiple factors should be considered to determine what a child or an adolescent needs to be told including age, cognitive and emotional maturity. Prior to offering any information, a health professional should gather together a general picture of the way the family thinks about HIV and its means of communication by posing three questions:

1. What have the parents or caregivers already told the child about his/her HIV infection?
2. What are the child's own representations and fantasies of the infection or disease, his/her level of understanding, his/her fears and questions about it?
3. Depending on the answers to 1 and 2, would the disclosure of HIV/AIDS diagnosis benefit the child and help him/her cope better with his/her health situation?

When a child asks for the name of the disease, it may be a clue that the child now understands what is happening and an indication of readiness to share his awareness. This is a "crucial" time for the adolescent which requires planning, anticipation and time. As a result, appropriate and consensual dialogue should take place in order to establish the individual pathways and steps of the disclosure process. When parents are reluctant to consider any kind of disclosure the reasons why it is worth telling the child or the adolescent a few things about his symptoms, pains and treatment should be actively discussed. Previously unresolved traumatic events may underlay this attitude and may need to be addressed. (Funck-Brentano, 1995).

In some cases of non disclosure health carers may sometimes notice non-verbal indirect signs that the adolescent understands what is going on. Health carers may interprete the message as a demand for naming the disease and talking about it, when the adolescent is just sharing his knowledge and does not appeal any verbal feedback. Instead, health carers' may receive the message and comply with this "half-spoken" level of communication in order to maintain the quality of the child-parent relationship. If the carers were to break this rule of silence, the parents may be upset or marginalised.

Experience shows that in families where parents are not able to support their children's awareness of the link between their symptoms and AIDS diagnosis, then denial of these links by the parents determine what the child or adolescent thinks or says about the disease for a very long time. Once the parents have missed the opportunity of disclosing minimal and honest information, then they have a hard time getting another opportunity to do so. Children may be embarrassed and protect their parents by avoiding thinking about or asking questions about their health. In the meantime this avoidance offers them the benefit of the doubt which in turn operates as an indispensable protection for some of them.

Disclosure is indeed required, but it is not always a priority. Sometimes there are indications that things have to be told. At other times, a period of latency is indicated. Close collaboration is therefore highly necessary.

With respect to prevention of sexual transmission, this concern has to be handled carefully and should not be the only factor to influence disclosure. Full disclosure of an AIDS diagnosis for the purpose of relieving parents from their fears is rather irrelevant when adolescents are clearly not yet pubescent or are still too immature to become sexually active. However, the issue should be discussed with the parents to enable them to teach their children about the general dangers they may be exposed to, AIDS being included in the list of sexually transmitted diseases. In addition, communities are making efforts to participate in adolescents' sexual education, schools are providing special sessions about it while automatic condom dispensers are displayed inside public schools.

CONCLUSION

Currently our experience with HIV infected adolescents is still limited as few children have so far reached adolescence. The coming years should broaden our knowledge of major issues regarding development, socialization and adolescents' abilities to attain adulthood. Indeed, in the future critical questions need to be researched more deeply regarding the long term impact of parental illness and loss, and the impact of HIV infection on adolescents, many of whom have experienced disruptive child rearing which might itself be detrimental to their personality development. Will past exposures disturb the adolescent's sense of security? Will they be of benefit or injury to their self-esteem and their sense of self-worth as a human being? Will the children and adolescents be provided with appropriate nurture and good models for identification, which they can internalize? Since sexual relationships and death concept might be strongly associated in their mind in reference to their parents' past experience, what will the effects be on their sexual life and desire to make children?

REFERENCES

Armstrong, D., Siedel, J., Swales, T. (1993) Pediatric HIV infection: a neuropsychological and educational challenge. *Journal of Learning Disabilities.* **26**, 92-103.

Bibace, R., Walsh, M.E. (1980) Development of children's concepts of illness. *Pediatrics,* **66**, 912-917

Blanche, S., Tardieu, M., Duliège, A.M. (1990) "Longitudinal study of 94 symptomatic infants with maternofoetal HIV infection: evidence for a bimodal expression of clinical and biological symptoms. *American Journal of Diseases of Children.* **144**, 1210-1215.

Blanche, S., Mayaux, M.J., Veber, F. *et al.* (1996) Separation between HIV-positive women and their children: The French Prospective Study, 1986 through 1993. *American Journal of Public Health.* **86**: 376-381.

Bose, S., Moss, H.A., Brouwers, P. *et al.* (1994) Psychologic adjustment of Human Immunodeficiency Virus-infected school-age children. *Developmental and Behavioral Pediatrics.* **15**, 26-33.

Brewster, A.B. (1982) Chronically ill hospitalized children's concepts of their illness. *Pediatrics.* **69**, 355-362

Brown, L.K., Schultz, R.J., Gragg, R.A., (1995) HIV-infected adolescents with haemophilia: adaptation and coping. *Pediatrics.* **96**, 459-463

Cadman. D., Boyle, M., Szatmari, P., Offord, D.R. (1987) Chronic illness, disability, and mental and social well-being: findings on the Ontario Child Health Study. *Pediatrics.* **79**, 805-813

Cohen, S., Mundy, T., Karassik, B. *et al.* (1991) Neuropsychological functioning in Human Immunodeficiency Virus type 1 seropositive children infected through neonatal blood transfusion. *Pediatrics.* **88**, 58-68.

Cohen, F.L. (1994) Research on families and pediatric Human Immunodeficiency Virus disease: a review and needed directions. *Developmental and Behavioral Pediatrics.* **15**, 34-41

Colegrove, R.W., Huntzinger, R.M. (1994) Academic, behavioral, and social adaptation of boys with Hemophilia/HIV disease. *Journal of Pediatric Psychology.* **19**, 457-473

Diamond, G., (1989) Developmental problems in children with HIV infection. *Mental Retardation.* **27**, 213-219.

Funck-Brentano, I. (1996) Aspects psychologiques de la prise en charge de l'enfant infecté par le VIH *Annales de Pediatric.*

Funck-Brentano, I. (1994) Les informations données à l'enfant sur son infection ou sa maladie. In: Droits de I'enfant et infection par le VIH. IDEF. Paris. 198-221.

Funck-Brentano, I. (1995) L'information de l'enfant sur sa maladie dans un cas d'infection à VIH: Parole et sens. *Psychiatrie de l'enfant.* XXXVII, **1**, 109-139.

Funck-Brentano, I. (in press) Troubles psychiatriques des enfants infectés par le VIH, *Journal du Sida,* 1997.

Funck-Brentano I. *et al.* (in press). SIDA et prise en charge nutritionnelle de l'enfant: enjeux psychologiques. In: Melchior J.C., Goulet O. Nutrition et SIDA. Masson. 1997.

Goulet O. *et al.* (in press). Prise en charge nutritionnelle an cours du VIH chez l'enfant. In: Melchior J.C., Goulet O. Nutrition et SIDA. Masson. 1997

Hardy, S.M., Armstrong, F.D., Routh, D.K. *et al.* (1994) Coping and communication among parents and children with Immunodeficiency Virus and Cancer. *Developmental and Behavioral Pediatrics*, **15**, 49-53.

Havens, J.F., Whitaker, A.H., Feldman, J.F., Ehrhardt, A.A. (1994) Psychiatric morbidity in school-age children with congenital Human Immunodeficiency Virus infection : a pilot study. *Developmental and Behavioral Pediatrics.* **15**, 18-25

Levenson, R.L., Mellins, C.A., Zawardzki, R., Kairam, R., Stein, Z. (1992). Cognitive assessment of Human Immunodeficiency Virus-exposed children. *AJDC.* **146**, 1479-1483

Lipson, M. (1993) What do you say to a child with AIDS? *Hastings Center Report* **23**, 6-12.

Lipson, M. (1994) Disclosure of diagnosis to children with Human Immunodeficiency Virus or Acquired Immunodeficiency Syndrome. *Developmental and Behavioral Pediatrics.* **15**, 61-65

Mellins, C.A., Levenson, R., Zawadzki, R. (1994) Effects of pediatrics HIV infection and prenatal drug exposure on mental and psychomotor development. *Journal of Pediatric Psychology.* **19**, 617-628.

Mellins, C.A, Enhardt, A.A. (1994) Families affected by pediatric Acquired Immunodeficiency Syndrome: sources of stress and coping. *Developmental and Behavioral Pediatrics.* **15**, 54-60

Papola, P., Alvarez, M., Cohen. H.J. (1994) Developmental and service needs of school-age children with Human Immunodeficiency Virus infection: a descriptive study. *Pediatrics.* **94**, 914-918

Perrin, E.C., Sayer, A.G., Willett, J.B. (1991) Sticks and stones may brake my bones... Reasoning, about illness causality and body functioning in children who have a chronic illness. *Pediatrics.* **88**, 608-619

Springer, K. (1994) Beliefs about illness causality among preschoolers with cancer : Evidence against immanence justice. *Journal of Pediatric Psychology.* **19**, 91-101

Tardieu, M., Mayaux, M.J., Seibel, N. *et al.* (1995) Cognitive assessment of school-age children infected with maternally transmitted Human Immunodeficiency Virus type 1. *Journal of Pediatrics.* **126**, 375-379

Tardieu, M. (in press), Neurological aspects of HIV1 infection in children, in Major problems in Neurology. London: Academic Press 1997.

Thompson, R.J., Hodges, K., Hamlet, K.W., (1989) A matched comparison of adjustment in children with cystic fibrosis and psychiatrically referred and nonreferred children. *Journal of Pediatric Psychology.* **15**, 745-759

Thompson, R.J., Gufstafson, K.E., Hamlett, K.W., Spock, A. (1992) Psychological adjustment of children with cystis fibrosis: the role of child cognitive processes and maternal adjustment. *Journal of Pediatric Psychology.* **17**, 741-755

Walsh, M.E., Bibace, R. (1991) Children's conceptions of AIDS: A developmental analysis. *Journal of Pediatric Psychology.* **16**, 273-285

Wiener, L., Theut, S., Steinberg, S., Riekert, K., Pizzo, P. (1994) The HIV infected child : parental responses and psychosocial implications. *American Journal of Orthopsychiatry.* **64**, 485-492.

12

The Medical Management of AIDS in Adolescents

BARRY S. PETERS & ANN REID

INTRODUCTION AND GENERAL PRINCIPLES

In this chapter we will discuss those conditions occurring in HIV infection and AIDS, and their treatment. We will then describe the therapies used against HIV itself and will include potential future treatments as well as current strategies.

Before considering specific issues of the medical management of HIV infection, however, it is important to grasp some general principles. These are:

Access to medical care

Probably the single most important factor in the medical management of patients with HIV infection is access to care. The provision of good access for different patient groups will allow diagnoses to be made and care to be delivered at the earliest possible stage. For example, most patients, when they are diagnosed with PCP (a pneumonia common in AIDS - see below) will receive similar and appropriate treatment; however, those patients who present late have a much worse prognosis than those patients who access medical care early on in their illness. Adolescents, along with certain ethnic minorities, are one of the "special groups" where access is even more crucial. Traditional models of care for HIV infection are not always appropriate for adolescents. They may, for example, refrain from attending the "adult" clinics. It is important that the means of delivering health care to this group is designed with their particular needs in mind.

Individualising health care

As well as differences between groups, there are obviously great differences in the needs of various patients within each group. With a chronic illness like AIDS it is important that a model of care is proposed that the patient might at least follow. This might not strictly be the best model of care for his health, but it will be a pragmatic one that he will accept because he has been involved with its design, and it is appropriate to his lifestyle. Failure to recognise the importance of this principle has meant that many adult patients have needlessly rejected the package of care offered to them. For adolescents we must be even more diligent in ensuring that the approach to care is right for them as an individual.

Constantly reassess the advantages and disadvantages of the current model of care

A recent article on the drug toxicities associated with treatments for HIV infection stated:

"With AIDS it is important to regard the prescriber's pen as another organ system which can be associated with morbidity and mortality, and which needs examining like any other for conditions that can be treated" (Peters *et al.*, 1994).

Similarly, all interventions, be they drugs, psychological care or social support, need reviewing regularly for every patient. This principle is even more important for the rapidly changing world of the adolescent.

SPECIFIC MANAGEMENT ISSUES

Clinical features of HIV infection and AIDS

AIDS is a result of prolonged infection with HIV. In 1982, the Centres for Disease Control laid down the definition of AIDS, and also classified HIV infection into a series of stages, or groups. The "CDC classifications" has been revised and added to several times over the years, and we will present the main points from the most recent (1993) revision.

The first stage of HIV infection, known as CDC Group I, is when people first become infected with the virus. The serum samples taken from blood of people becoming infected show an important change. Before infection with HIV the serum does not show HIV antibodies, or the "HIV antibody test is negative". Within a few weeks to a few months of becoming infected, the body produces antibodies to HIV, which show up in the serum, and the person will now show a "positive HIV antibody test". This process of changing from uninfected with a negative test to infected with a positive test is known as "seroconversion" (De Jong *et al.*, 1991). Usually the person feels well during this process, and there is nothing to suspect that he has become infected. In approximately 20% of cases there is an accompanying illness. This "seroconversion illness" may resemble glandular fever, and so the person may have enlarged glands in the neck or elsewhere, a skin rash, and feel weak or flu-like (Hoover *et al.*, 1993). The symptoms of acute seroconversion illness might be much milder, or as mentioned above might be absent. Occasionally, the symptoms are very severe, with a meningo-encephalititis with drowsiness or unconsciousness.

The importance of identifying when seroconversion took place for an individual person is that it gives them a guide to prognosis and when they might expect to develop disease. If the date of seroconversion is unknown, then there are no tests which will give an accurate idea of how long that individual has been infected. One can only assume that infection occurred no later than their last possible risk factor for contracting HIV.

Following acute infection, the next stage, Group 2, is one of asymptomatic infection. During this stage the patient is infected with the virus, but has no outward signs of disease, and looks and feels normal. This stage lasts on average for approximately ten years, but can vary from two years or less up to 15 years or more. It is not known at this stage whether some people will remain asymtomatic forever, or whether everyone infected with HIV will eventually develop AIDS. There are however, a significant minority of patients who remain symptom-free for well beyond the average length of time. These "slow progressors" or "non-progressors" are being studied to see if they will yield vital clues to how the immune system controls HIV infection. It is almost unheard of for someone who is infected with HIV to clear the infection and become HIV antibody negative. Although there are a few unsubstantiated, at the time of writing, there is only one well-documented case of this occurring, and that was in a child. Therefore, once someone becomes infected with HIV, they remain both infected, and infectious to others, for the rest of their life.

Some patients, about one fifth, pass through a third stage of HIV infection, where the lymph glands throughout the body become swollen for 3 months or more, and there is weight loss and constitutional symptoms such as fever. This stage, known as Group 3 disease, is "persistent generalised lymphadenopathy" (or "PGL"). The lymph nodes eventually shrink back to their normal size and the patients become asymptomatic again, although once they have been classified as Group 3, they never go back to a previous group.

The final stage of HIV infection is Group 4 disease, and is comprised of the various diseases which occur with advancing immunosuppression. Pre-AIDS or ARC (AIDS-related complex) are older terms that are still in use and refer to a stage of HIV infection that is milder than AIDS. Examples of these conditions are oral candidiasis (thrush in the mouth), Hairy Oral Leukoplakia (HOL), and seborrhoeic dermatitis. Patients do not necessarily present with these less severe manifestations of HIV disease, and their first sign of illness might be one of the more severe AIDS-defining diseases. This is a very important point, because it is possible for someone to have advanced immunosuppression whilst still feeling well and without any symptoms at all. This is one argument for identifying individuals who might be at risk of being infected with HIV, so that their health can be monitored, treatment can be offered and they can make appropriate plans for the future.

AIDS represents the final stages of HIV infection, but even so the prognosis and the quality of life can vary greatly between individuals. Hence, following an AIDS diagnosis, some people continue to survive for many years with a good quality of life, whereas others might suffer from severe disability, rapid decline and early death. Many patients with AIDS are well enough to continue life with few restrictions for several years, and if they chose to do so, to remain at work. The average survival from a diagnosis of AIDS is between 2 to 3 years, but depends largely on the HIV-related conditions the person has suffered from (Peters *et al.*, 1991).

Conditions which define someone as having AIDS belong to several categories:

Opportunistic infections

Tumours

Effects of HIV on the nervous system

Certain systemic or general conditions

Opportunistic infections

An opportunistic infection is one that would not normally occur in a healthy individual with an intact immune system; it needs the right opportunity, for example the weakened immune system resulting from HIV infection.

There are conditions other than HIV infection that can weaken the body's ability to fight infection and lead to opportunistic infections, e.g., other immunodeficiency diseases, advanced malignancy, diabetes and patients receiving immunosuppressive drugs to reduce the probability of rejection of transplanted organs. Hence, before AIDS is diagnosed in someone, it is wise to consider the possibility of these other conditions, and ensure a positive HIV antibody test result is known; if the person declines an HIV test then it is important to ensure that sufficient risk factor(s) are present before assuming an AIDS condition.

There are 3 stages in the treatment of opportunistic infections in HIV disease, prophylaxis (preventative treatment), active treatment if the infection occurs, and maintenance therapy to prevent reactivation of the infection. Prophylaxis is not always possible or desirable, but it is most useful when a safe and effective oral drug exists for a common and severe opportunistic infection. This is the case with prophylaxis for PCP (see below). Until a means is found to restore the immune function of someone with AIDS, those opportunistic infections that are successfully treated will probably reoccur. Maintenance therapy is therefore required to reduce the likelihood of repeated infection.

The opportunistic infections that occur in AIDS are as follows:

Pneumocystis carinii pneumonia (PCP) – This is one of the commonest opportunistic infections that occurs in AIDS (Peters *et al.*, 1991). It can range from a very mild to a very severe or fatal chest infection, depending upon how early the condition is recognised and treated (Hughes, 1992). The early recognition and treatment of this condition is one of the reasons why the average survival of patients with AIDS has increased over time. Most cases of PCP occur when there is at least moderate immunosuppression (CD4 count < 250 mm^3). Therefore when the CD4 count has fallen to this level, patients should be offered prophylaxis against PCP. The best form of prophylaxis is cotrimoxazole (Septrin/Bactrim) tablets, but if an allergy develops to these then alternatives, such as pentamidine solution via a nebuliser, can be used.

The treatment of PCP depends on the severity at presentation. If the patient has a severe chest infection with hypoxia then urgent admission and treatment with intravenous cotrimoxazole and intravenous steroids is required. If the patient presents with a mild chest infection due to PCP then he can often be treated as an outpatient with oral medication. The crucial management issue with PCP, for both doctors and patients is: PCP should always be suspected in an HIV positive individual who has respiratory symptoms, even mild symptoms such as a dry cough or slight shortness of breath. If neglected, early mild PCP can progress from an easily treatable condition to a severe pneumonia that can prove fatal (Brenner *et al.*, 1987).

Hence it is crucial that adolescents infected with HIV have easy access to appropriate medical services so that they can receive prompt diagnosis and treatment of PCP or other opportunistic conditions at an early stage.

Toxoplasmosis – the commonest site for this infection in a person with AIDS is the brain, and the patients might develop fits or paralysis due to brain damage.

As with PCP, a fairly good treatment exists for this condition, and therefore early diagnosis is important. A CT brain scan will usually show the typical lesions. Maintenance therapy is essential for this condition.

Cytomegalovirus – a virus that is common in the general population and even more so in male homosexuals. It remains dormant until the severe immunosuppression associated with AIDS reactivates the organism. The most common site affected by cytomegalovirus is the eye, where involvement of the retina can lead to blindness (Jabs *et al.*, 1989). The bowel is the next commonest site to be involved, with resulting colitis.

Treatment for cytomegalovirus disease has in the past meant intravenous administration of the drugs ganciclovir or foscarnet in hospital followed by lifelong maintenance intravenous therapy. This maintenance therapy required the insertion of an indwelling catheter, and this carried the risk of infection, was often inconvenient and was cosmetically undesirable. An oral form of ganciclovir has recently been introduced for maintenance therapy, and appears to be a successful alternative to intravenous ganciclovir.

Cryptoccal meningitis – Cryptococcus neoformans is a fungal infection that can cause meningitis in people with HIV, and although treatment is available, and the patient might recover initially, the prognosis following this infection is poor. If cryptococcal meningitis is suspected then it is necessary to perform a lumbar puncture to look for the presence of the fungus in the cerebrospinal fluid. Treatment options include intravenous or oral fluconazole, and intravenous amphotericin B. Amphotericin B is a toxic drug and needs careful monitoring to prevent side-effects such as renal failure. A new form of amphotericin B, liposomal amphotericin B, is much less toxic and represents an advance in management.

PML – Progressive multifocal encephalopathy

This is a viral infection that causes a mass within the brain substance, similar to a brain tumour. PML usually responds poorly to treatment and carries a bad prognosis.

Cryptosporidium – This is an organism that might cause mild diarrhoea in the general population, but can cause severe diarrhoea and malnutrition in people with HIV. Cryptosporidium bowel disease is often refractory to any form of treatment in patients who are immunosuppressed.

Candida (Thrush) infection of the oesophagus – Candida albicans is a fungus infection that manifests itself frequently in the general population, and vulvo-vaginal candidiasis is common in healthy women. Candida infection of the mouth, most typically presenting as white plaques, or of the oesophagus, is associated with a wide range of conditions, such as diabetes, the use of antibiotics, ill-fitting dentures, malnourishment etc., as well as HIV infection. In mild or moderate immunosuppression candida might be confined to the mouth, but with the severe immunosuppression of AIDS it can affect the oesophagus, causing severe pain on swallowing. Oral or oesophageal candida is easily treated when it first presents, but over time, the fungus can become much more refractory to first line medication.

Tuberculosis involving at least one site outside the lungs. Tuberculosis has enjoyed a resurgence as a result of the HIV pandemic (Johnson and Chaisson 1994). Multi-drug-resistant strains of Mycobacterium tuberculosis have occurred in HIV - infected individuals (Dooley *et al.*, 1992). Some of the health care workers managing these patients have contracted this strain of TB, and a few have subsequently died. Good compliance with drug therapy is thought to be important in preventing the emergence of resistant strains. Lifelong maintenance therapy with at least one drug is usually offered to patients to prevent further episodes

"MAC" or "MAI" Mycobacterium avium complex/ Mycobacterium avium intracellulare - Both these terms refer to an organism that resembles the one which causes tuberculosis. MAC, however, is rare unless the patient has very advanced immunosuppression (CD4 count < 100 mm^3); at this stage of immunosuppression, MAC becomes common. Many of the features of MAC infection are non-specific, such as lethargy, fever, or anaemia. Drugs exist for the prophylaxis and treatment of MAC, but each patient needs to be assessed individually as these drugs are frequently toxic. It is important to regularly compare the benefits of treatment to the adverse effects.

Recurrent bacterial pneumonias are unusual in healthy young people; the occurence of two "bacteriologically proven" cases in a 12 month period signifies that an HIV infected individual has a severe enough immunodeficiency to be classified as having AIDS. The commonest cause of these pneumonias is the organism *Streptococcus pneumoniae*, and hence many practitioners offer prophylactic pneumococcal vaccination to people with HIV infection.

Recurrent salmonella septicaemia Septicaemia on more than one occasion caused by the bowel pathogen Salmonella equates with an AIDS diagnosis. The symptoms might be those of gastroenteritis, with diarrhoea and abdominal pain and occasionally frankly bloody stools, or the patient might have no bowel symptoms, but just be "severely ill" and shocked due to septicaemia. If suspected then the disease is usually easily treated with intravenous fluids and the appropriate antibiotics.

HIV encephalopathy Direct infection of the brain with HIV can lead to a deterioration in mental function. CT scans of the brain reveal thinning of the cerebral cortex. An alternative name for this condition, particularly when it is severe, is "AIDS dementia complex". There is some suggestion that patients taking zidovudine have a lower incidence of this condition, and indeed patients with HIV encephalopathy often improve following treatment with relatively high dose zidovudine.

Other AIDS defining conditions not mentioned above include, persistent herpes simplex virus infections, and diseases uncommon in the UK, such as histoplasmosis and isosporiasis.

The use of a low CD4 count (less than 200mm^3) to define AIDS has been adopted by the USA and some other countries, but not currently by Europe.

AIDS in Africa often presents differently to AIDS in the western world, and to reflect this, and the often reduced diagnostic facilities available, there are several differences in the criteria used to define AIDS in Africa.

AIDS in infants presents a different clinical picture to AIDS in adults, and hence there is a separate classification system in use for this age group.

Tumours occurring in patients with AIDS

There are 3 tumours that are common in advanced HIV infection and are AIDS diagnoses (Milliken & Boyle, 1993).

Kaposi's sarcoma usually presents first as a red or purplish plaque on the skin, but it can also affect the internal organs such as the lungs or bowel. Kaposi's sarcoma associated with AIDS is much commoner in patients who acquire HIV via the sexual route, and even in this group is much commoner in men. This tumour occurs, for example, in about one third of male homosexuals, in contrast to intravenous drug users or patients infected via blood products, where it is found in only 1-2%.

Kaposi's sarcoma often responds well to treatment in the early stages, for example with chemotherapy of radiotherapy. Interferon-alpha can be very effective in early stage AIDS-KS but the side-effects usually mitigate against its use. Local radiotherapy to cutaneous lesions may produce a very good response, and can prove of great cosmetic benefit. Lesions not responding to this therapy can often be camouflaged with make-up.

Extensive disease, particularly "internal involvement" of e.g., the lungs or the bowel, usually leads to death within months. In this situation chemotherapy may reduce the tumour load and improve the quality of life.

Lymphomas – Certain types of lymphoma, that is the high grade non-Hodgkin's B-cell lymphomas, are found fairly commonly in people with AIDS. The outlook following diagnosis of this tumour is usually poor. If the patient is fit enough, then a course of chemotherapy and/or radiotherapy might improve symptoms and prolong survival.

Cervical carcinoma – This tumour has only recently been added to the list of AIDS defining conditions. It is important that women infected with HIV undergo cervical smears for cytology screening at frequent intervals, e.g., every 6 months, in order that any neoplastic changes are detected at an early and curable stage (Maiman *et al.*, 1990).

Antiviral Treatment for HIV

The "Life Cycle" of HIV infection of a cell is complex. A simplified scheme of this cycle is given in figure 1 and we have marked the points where anti-HIV therapy has been targeted.

The ideal anti-HIV drug would be:

- non-toxic,
- prevent further HIV replication throughout the body,
- effective at all stages of HIV infection
- should be effective when taken orally and at widely spaced intervals, and
- HIV should not develop resistance to the drug over time.

With these principles in mind, let us look at the anti-HIV drugs licensed for use, and some that are showing promising results in clinical trials.

AZT (Zidovudine) and other reverse transcriptase inhibitors

Zidovudine is the most widely used anti-HIV drug and was the first such drug to gain a license. It began to be widely used in 1986 when a study showed that patients

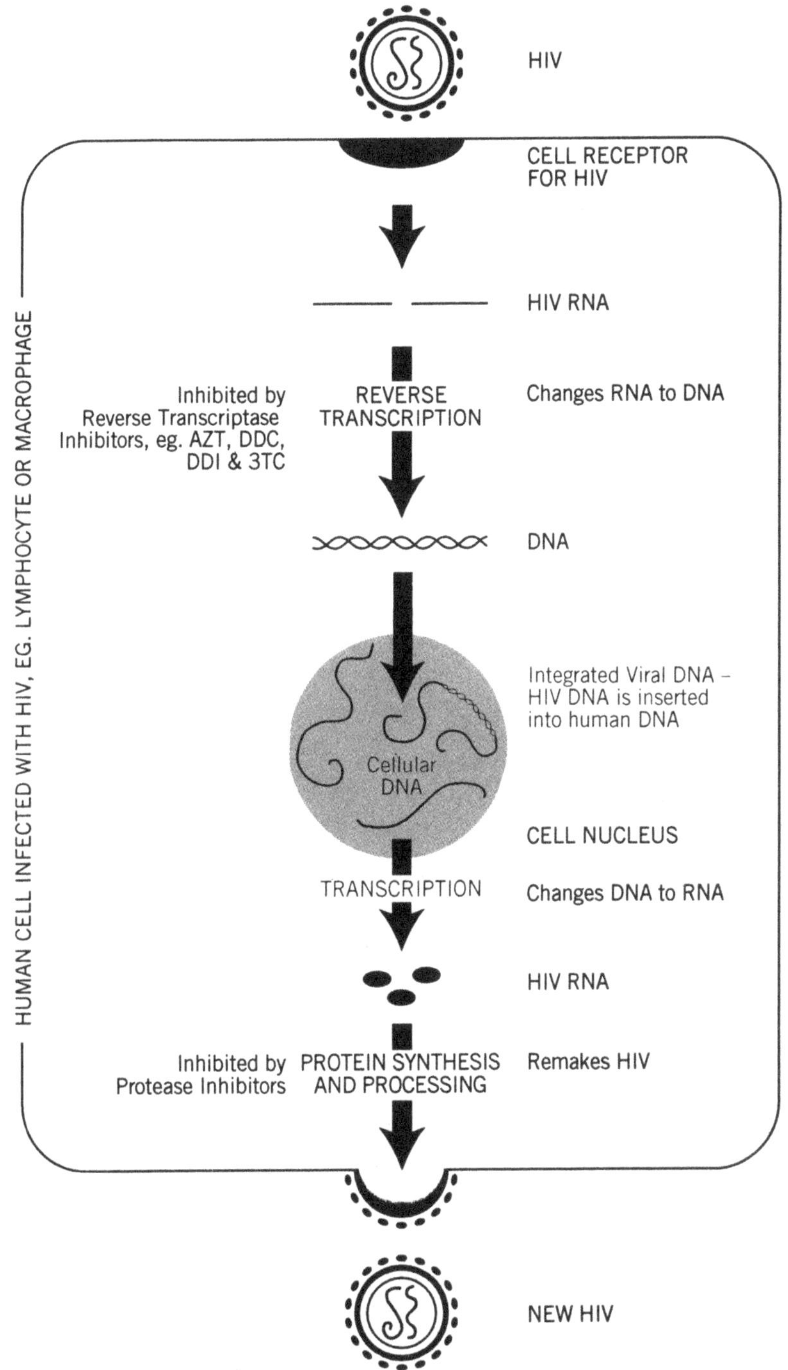

Fig. 1 Lifecycle of the Human Immunodeficiency Virus

with AIDS who took Zidovudine lived longer and had less opportunistic infections than patients who did not take the drug. (Fischl and Dickinson 1987). However, zidovudine is far from an ideal drug for several reasons. It has toxicity in a proportion of patients, for example, bone marrow toxicity leading to anaemia, reduced numbers of platelets (thrombocytopenia) leading to bleeding, and reduction in neutrophils (neutropenia - reduction in a type of white cell, not usually affected in HIV disease, that helps protect against certain microbes) leading to infection. Furthermore the Anglo-French "Concorde" study demonstrated that Zidovudine has no long-term benefit on the survival of patients who are asymptomatic when they took the drug (Concorde Coordinating Committee 1994). Over time the predominant HIV strains in any individual taking zidovudine become resistant to the drug; this development of resistance is probably the main reason why zidovudine loses its effectiveness over time when used as sole treatment against HIV (i.e., used as monotherapy).

Zidovudine is similar to one of the nucleotides of DNA, and acts either by fitting into a DNA chain and terminating its further replication, and by inhibiting reverse transcriptase.

Three other reverse transcriptase inhibitors have been licensed by the middle of 1995, and they are also nucleoside analogues. These are DDC (zalcitabine/Hivid), DDI (didanosine/Videx) and D4T (stavudine/Zerit). Their use can be summarised as follows: there appear to be no clear advantages over zidovudine as monotherapy, but they have different side-effects and therefore are an alternative if intolerance to zidovudine occurs.

The future

The future will probably lie with drug combinations as these should have a synergistic antiviral action, reduced toxicity and reduced risk of emergence of drug-resistant virus. Several large clinical trials of combination therapy are already underway. As well as the licensed reverse transcriptase inhibitors, there is a new generation of potentially promising drugs and therapeutic approaches. 3TC (Lamivudine) is a reverse transcriptase inhibitor which has shown some encouraging results when used with zidovudine. There are several non-nucleoside reverse transcriptase inhibitors that are under development, e.g. loviride and nevirapine. Protease inhibitors interfere with the processing of viral proteins, and several of these compounds are in an advanced stage of human clinical trials. It seems strongly possible at this stage that a protease inhibitor will be one of the drugs used in combination therapy against HIV.

There are several other potential targets of HIV replication (see figure). In addition, there are other approaches under development, such as immuno-therapeutic vaccination. This strategy involves immunising an HIV positive individual with a component of HIV in order to provoke a beneficial immune response. Another strategy is gene therapy whereby some of the genes of HIV are altered so that the pathogenicity of the virus is reduced or prevented.

Management issues of particular relevance to adolescents

There are many aspects of the management of HIV infection and AIDS which can be improved for the adolescent population.

Suitability of clinics

Adolescents fall between two stools. They are too old for the paediatric clinics, and too young for the adult clinics. They often suffer much unease when they attend clinics outside their age group. In addition, many adolescents initially attend paediatric clinics only to be transferred later to the adult services. These factors often lead to either failure of attendance or late utilisation of services. As we have already discussed, if a patient presents early with his symptoms, then he is much more likely to make a good response to therapy.

It would be ideal to have designated "adolescent clinics", in the same way that several districts have special clinics for haemophiliacs, intravenous drug users, "working women", lesbians and gay men. If there are very few adolescents with HIV in a particular district, then it is difficult to justify the resources for such clinics. Much can still be done to achieve the aims of a specialised clinic, which is to offer the adolescent treatment away from adults, at a time that is suitable for them (usually in the early evening) and from staff with appropriate skills. If a designated clinic is not possible, then an hour can be set aside after another clinic on a regular basis, or special arrangements can be made to see adolescents in a more private setting. Currently there are few districts that have "age appropriate" sexual health or AIDS clinics for adolescents; for those that do, their value is recognised by user and provider alike.

Clinical trials and adolescents

There are no large studies looking at drug therapies among adolescents with HIV. Indeed, in many countries those below a certain age are usually excluded from adult trials. In the UK this exclusion usually applies to those under 18 years. In this respect adolescents are similar to women in that they are often denied the possible therapeutic benefits that trials of promising compounds might bring. Furthermore, any differences in treatment responses between adolescents and older age groups are not being studied.

Different prescribing requirements for adolescents

Regimens that might be acceptable to many adults, might be inappropriate for the teenager, particular those attending school or college. For example, multiple dosing regimens that require drugs to be taken when at school highlight the person's illness, particularly when the school insists in dispensing the medication of its pupils. Therefore every effort should be made to have no more than a twice daily dosing schedule for long-term medication. As well as reducing stigma, it will also improve compliance. Once or twice daily medication can be achieved for most situations. For instance, newer compounds for use against the viruses which cause herpes ulceration and shingles, valacyclovir and famciclovir, have a much longer half-life than acyclovir.

REFERENCES

Brenner, M., Ognibene, F.P., Lack, E.E. *et al.* (1987) Prognostic factors and life expectancy of patients with Acquired Immunodeficiency Syndrome and pneumocystis carinii pneumonia. *Am Rev Respir Dis.* 1199 - 1206.

Centres for Disease Control, (1993). Revised classification system for HIV infection and expanded surveillance case definition for AIDS among adolescents and adults. *J Am Med Assoc.* **269**, 729-730.

Concorde Co-ordinating Committee: MRC/ANRS. (1994) Randomised, double-blind placebo-controlled trial of immediate and deferred zidovudine in symptom-free HIV infection. *Lancet.* **343**, 871-881.

De Jong, M.D., Hulseboch, H.J., Lange, J.M.A. (1991) Clinical, virological and immunological features of primary HIV-I infection. *Genitourinary Med.* **67**, 367-373.

Dooley, S.W., Jarvis, W.R., Martone, W.J., Snider, D.E. (1992) Multi-drug resistant tuberculosis. *Ann Intern Med.* **117**, 257-259.

Fischl, M.A., Richman, D.D., Grieco, M.H. *et al.* (1987). The efficacy of Azidothymidine (AZT) in the treatment of patients with AIDS and AIDS-related complex. *N Engl J Med.* **317**, 185-191.

Hoover, D.R., Saah, A.J., Bacellar, H. *et al.* (1993) Signs and symptoms of "asymptomatic" HIV-I infection in homosexual men. *J AIDS.* **6**, 66-71

Hughes, W.T. (1992) Pneumocystis carinii infection: an update; *Medicine* (Baltimore). **5**, 175-178.

Jabs, D.A., Green, W.R., Fox, R., Polk, F., Bartlett, J.G. (1989). Ocular manifestations of acquired immune deficiency syndrome. *Opthalmology.* **96**, 1092-1099.

Johnson, M.P., Chaisson, R.E. (1994). Tuberculosis and HIV Disease. In AIDS Clinical Review 1993/1994, Volberding, P., Jacobson, M.A. (Eds.), Publ. Marcel Dekker, New York.

Maiman, M., Fruchter, R.G., Serur, E. *et al.* (1990). Human immunodeficiency virus infection and cervical neoplasia. *Gynecol Oncol.* **38**, 377-382.

Milliken, S., Boyle, M.J. (1993) Update on HIV and neoplastic disease. *AIDS.* **7**, S203-209.

Peters, B.S., Beck, E.J., Coleman, D.G. *et al.* (1991) Changing disease patterns in people with AIDS in a referral centre in the United Kingdom: the changing face of AIDS. *BMJ* **302**, 203-207.

Peters, B.S., Carlin., E, Weston, R.J. *et al.* (1994) Adverse effects of drugs used in the management of opportunistic infections associated with HIV infection. B. Peters. *et al.* *Drug Safety*, **10**, 439-454.

13

Looking Forward: Future Directions for Prevention of HIV among Adolescents

RALPH J. DiCLEMENTE

INTRODUCTION

Behaviour change remains the only practical strategy for the primary prevention of HIV. Thus, there is an overriding urgency to develop and implement behavioural interventions which motivate adolescents to adopt and maintain HIV- preventive practices; particularly condom use during sexual intercourse. While modifying adolescents' sexual behaviour poses formidable challenges, there is accumulating empirical data indicating that increasing condom use is an achievable goal.

Many facets of the HIV epidemic among adolescents have been described in previous chapters. This chapter, unlike its predecessors, attempts to discern fruitful directions for future prevention efforts. In particular, this chapter examines potentially new and important programmatic considerations that may enhance prevention efforts. Amplification of programmatic efficacy in future HIV prevention may be contingent on the adequacy with which each of the following elements prove efficacious, can be incorporated into interventions, and can be tailored to the socio-cultural contextual environments of different adolescent subgroups. To facilitate an appreciation of these intervention elements, it is useful to briefly trace the genealogy of HIV prevention intervention programmes for adolescents and observe their evolution over the course of the epidemic.

Design of Effective Sexual Behaviour Modification Interventions: A Historical Perspective

Behavioural interventions, designed to reduce adolescents' HIV- associated risk behaviours, have evolved slowly over the course of the epidemic. Indeed, it wasn't until the mid-eighties that adolescents were even considered a population at-risk of HIV infection (DiClemente, Zorn & Temoshok, 1986) and the first wave of interventions initiated. Initially, the first generation of HIV prevention interventions focused primarily on increasing adolescents' knowledge of HIV and emphasizing the risk and consequences of disease. These interventions were predicated on a fundamental premise; namely, that if youth had greater knowledge about HIV and its association with sexual intercourse, and the consequences of HIV infection (i.e., AIDS and consequently, debilitation and death), they would rationally choose to avoid unprotected intercourse. Unfortunately, these prevention programmes were hastily developed and implemented. Few included an underlying theoretical model that conceptualized adolescents' sexual behaviour and decision-making based on well-defined psychological principles of behaviour. Moreover, politicalization of the HIV epidemic severely constrained the ability of programme planners with regard to utilizing a broader range of risk-reduction techniques and strategies to motivate adolescents' adoption of safer sex practices. In general, this generation of HIV interventions, though well-intentioned, was not effective at promoting adolescents to modify HIV risk behaviours.

The next generation of HIV- prevention interventions included considerable knowledge content, but did not give as much emphasis to the biology of HIV/AIDS and the biological consequences of infection. Instead, they devoted much more emphasis to values clarification and developing social competency skills, especially decision-making skills. The values clarification exercises were designed to help adolescents become clear about their basic values as well as their values about sexual behaviour. Health educators gave adolescents dilemmas to solve and discuss, but commonly did not emphasize that particular values were right or wrong. These programmes emphasized generic skills, such as the basic steps involved in making a decision. When these skills and values were applied to sexual issues, these programmes often spelled out the pros and cons of engaging in sexual intercourse. Proponents of this approach believed that if adolescents' values became more clear and their decision-making skills improved, then they would be more likely to avoid risk-taking behaviour.

Numerous studies have measured the impact of these first two generations of programmes upon the knowledge of adolescents and the findings from these studies are nearly unanimous – providing instruction in HIV did result in significant increases in knowledge of HIV and awareness of HIV- associated risk behaviours. However, it has become increasingly clear that increasing adolescents' knowledge about HIV is only weakly associated with decreasing their HIV- associated risk behaviours. Clearly, while HIV knowledge may be necessary, as a foundation to enhance understanding of the disease and transmission of the virus, it is not sufficient to motivate adolescents' adoption of HIV- preventive practices.

Empirical data derived primarily from recently completed observational cross-sectional and longitudinal cohort studies among diverse adolescent populations (DiClemente *et al.*, 1996; DiClemente, 1991; 1992; Joffe, 1993; Wight, 1992), identifying the determinants of high-risk behaviour and, more importantly, the determinants of safer sex behaviour have been integrated into the present generation of prevention programmes. In general, the present generation of HIV prevention programmes which are theory-driven, emphasize motivational factors, provide skills training, including partner communication, sexual negotiation, resistance skills, condom application skills, and that attempts to modify peer norms are more effective at promoting the adoption of HIV- preventive behaviours (Kelly & Murphy, 1992; Fisher & Fisher, 1992; Coates, 1990; Choi & Coates, 1994; DiClemente, 1993; Kirby & DiClemente, 1994; D'Angelo & DiClemente, 1996). These interventions have shown the capacity to reduce adolescents' HIV- associated risk behaviours. However, while demonstrating the ability to significantly enhance adolescents' adoption and use of HIV - preventive strategies, the magnitude of observed behavioural changes reported (i.e. programme effect sizes) have been, by and large, modest.

Future Intervention Research is Urgently Needed

While promising results have been observed, the effect sizes of behavioural intervention studies, although statistically significant, may not be comparably clinically significant. There is an important differentiation between statistical and clinical significance that is often times unclear. Thus, an intervention programme that reduces adolescents' HIV- associated risk behaviours may be statistically significant but may not markedly reduce adolescents' risk of HIV infection or impede, to any substantial degree, the spread of the HIV epidemic. For instance, many of the successful intervention studies (unfortunately, the number of unsuccessful intervention studies remains unknown) report relatively modest decrements in adolescents' risk behaviours. It is unclear that increasing adolescents' use of condoms by 10% or 15% will translate into a proportionate decrease in their risk for HIV infection. HIV infection, unlike many other chronic disease conditions, does not require cumulative exposures; a single exposure may result in infection triggering the pathological process which result in a loss of immunologic competence. Thus, it is unknown if there is a one-to-one relationship between decreasing adolescents' risk behaviours and decreasing their risk for HIV infection. Clearly, new and innovative intervention research is needed to amplify the effects of behaviour change programmes.

Directions for Future Intervention Research

To facilitate the development of a new generation of prevention interventions may require identifying new theoretical models on which to predicate behavioural interventions. In addition, new intervention modalities and strategies will need to be identified and rigorously evaluated to assess their effectiveness. Moreover, to reach a broader population, intervention research must begin to develop programmes that target the community rather than the individual. Furthermore, there is a need to disseminate existing intervention programmes that have already demonstrated programmatic efficacy while new and more effective programmes are under development. And finally, we need to discuss the role of public and health policy as a potential impediment or facilitator for the development and implementation of behavioural interventions. Each of these issues is considered in turn.

The Search for Models of Behaviour to Guiding the Development of HIV- preventive Programmes

High-risk sexual behaviour among adolescents is not random, uncontrollable, or inevitable. Many factors, both individual (intrapersonal) and social (interpersonal) contribute to an adolescents' propensity to engage in HIV- related sexual risk-taking. In essence, adolescents' sexual behaviour represents the behavioural endpoint of a multifactorial decision-making process that weighs a myriad of relevant internal and external influences; interpersonal, social, economic, psychological influences within a cultural context superimposed over traditions, values and patterns of social organization (DiClemente, 1992). Fortunately, many of these factors are modifiable. However, such a complex decision-making process is not likely to be understood in unidimensional or simplistic terms or, more importantly, be modified without addressing many of these influences. Therefore, utilizing a theoretical model that addresses the interplay between adolescents' cognitions, attitudes and beliefs, their behaviour and environmental influences, improves the likelihood of programmatic efficacy. One model of behaviour that has demonstrated its applicability for developing HIV prevention interventions for adolescents is Social Cognitive Theory.

Social Cognitive Theory

Social Cognitive Theory has proven particularly useful as a foundation for developing HIV risk-reduction interventions, especially for adolescents and multicultural populations. (Bandura, 1992, 1994). The cornerstones of this model include the provision of timely and accurate information, developing and mastering social competency skills through observational learning techniques (e.g., social modeling) and active learning techniques (e.g., role playing, preferably a series of graded-intensity of high-risk situations), enhancing self-efficacy to communicate assertively and effectively with sex partners and developing a supportive peer network to reinforce the maintenance of safer sex behaviours. Many effective prevention interventions for adolescents have been based on Social Cognitive Theory (D'Angelo & DiClemente, 1996). There are, however, emerging models of behaviour change that may also be applicable to modifying adolescents' risk behaviours. One particularly promising model is the Trans-theoretical Model.

Trans-theoretical Model of Behaviour Change: Applicability for HIV- prevention

The Transtheoretical Model of Behaviour Change (TMC) (Prochaska & DiClemente, C. 1983, 1984) is a relatively new model which includes elements of SCT as well as other models. The TMC defines behaviour change as an incremental, continuous, and a dynamic process. Thus, acquisition of new behaviour is the endpoint of a decision-making process in which adolescents progress through a sequence of specific stages. The TMC has been applied to a broad range of health-related behaviours including smoking cessation, exercise, adoption, diet, sun exposure, cocaine use, and contraceptive and condom use, adoption and continuation, suggesting that the underlying principles that facilitate change may be quite similar across a diversity of behaviours. However, while demonstrating its applicability for many of these health-related behaviours, the TMC remains largely untested in the area of sexual risk-reduction.

The TMC's four key constructs – stages of change, processes of change, decisional balance (pros and cons), and self-efficacy may be applicable to reducing adolescents' high-risk sexual behaviour. In addition, the TMC is a flexible, comprehensive and integrative model of behaviour change, able to incorporate new constructs such as sexual assertiveness in the model, enhancing the TMC's effectiveness for understanding sexual behaviour. Furthermore, another critical construct, particularly when examining adolescent sexual behaviour, is the influence of referent-group norms. Perceived peer norms is also discussed within the context of the TMC. Lastly, accumulating empirical evidence suggests that condom use behaviour is not uniform, but varies markedly depending on whether they are engaged in sexual intercourse with a primary partner or a non-primary (casual) partner. The TMC also addresses condom use behaviour with the two types of partners. Overall, the TMC provides a promising theoretical framework in which to develop and implement HIV- prevention interventions for adolescents; one that may be particularly useful for examining the reduction of high-risk sexual behaviours over time (Grimley, DiClemente, R., Prochaska, Riley, 1995).

Peer Advocacy Models: A Promising Intervention Strategy

Peer Advocacy Models (PAM), derived from Social Cognitive Theory, and based in developmental theory, recruit and train peers indigenous to a large target population to serve as leaders, educators and counsellors to become HIV- preventive behaviour change agents. Peer educators have been used effectively to prevent and, with less efficacy, to reduce adolescents' use of substances such as tobacco, alcohol and marijuana (Hansen & Graham, 1991; Klepp, Halper, & Perry, 1986; Perry & Grant, 1988; Robinson *et al.*, 1987; Botvin, 1986; Telch *et al.*, 1990). With respect to HIV- associated behaviours, PAM-based interventions in clinic-based risk-reduction studies have also demonstrated an ability to enhance HIV knowledge (Rickert, Jay & Gottlieb, 1991) and decrease risk behaviours Slap *et al.*, 1991). PAM-based behaviour change interventions, however, have not been extensively tested as an HIV- prevention strategy for adolescents.

Peer advocacy models offer a number of advantages over adult-led programmes when targeting interventions for adolescents. Peers may be more effective teachers of social skills, more influential models of health-promoting behaviour, and can serve as credible role models because they are members of the adolescents' social milieu. Peers can also help to change normative expectations about the frequency of the targeted behaviour in the peer group. Finally, peers can offer social support for performance of desired behaviours and for avoidance of health-damaging behaviours (DiClemente, 1993). These advantages are particularly important when educating adolescents in environments where social networks are limited and social norms, which may encourage and support risk-taking behaviour, are highly influential (DiClemente & Houston-Hamilton, 1989).

Several studies have successfully used peer-based models for reducing high-risk sexual behaviour in adult populations (Kelly *et al.*, 1991). However, peer interventions, such as the one developed by Slap and her colleagues (1992), are just now being evaluated with adolescents; particularly in countries most severely impacted by the HIV epidemic (Aggleton *et al.*, 1994). Perry and Sieving (1993) describe promising peer-led programmes designed to reach especially high-risk and hard-to-access populations of homeless and out-of-school adolescents. Although not yet published, available data indicate that peer leaders were positively perceived by other youth and were effective at communicating sexual risk-reduction messages and dispelling perceptions of high-risk sexual behaviour as normative. Clearly, peer involvement in the implementation of HIV prevention interventions warrants further consideration as one strategy for enhancing programmatic efficacy.

Health care providers as behaviour change agents: Windows of opportunity for HIV- prevention

While school and community-based prevention efforts are undoubtedly important in disseminating HIV prevention information, another critical, but underutilized access point for educating adolescents about HIV and other sexually transmitted diseases is during the provision of health care.

Pediatricians are most likely to be engaged in treating adolescents during the time of their onset of sexual and drug behaviours (American Academy of Pediatrics, 1990). Thus, clinical interactions between the pediatrician and adolescent patient become a window of opportunity to assess the prevalence of sexual and drug risk behaviours, evaluate the adolescent's physical and psychological maturation and provide developmentally-appropriate HIV prevention information (DiClemente & Brown, 1994). Unfortunately, there is ample data to indicate that this important channel of prevention information is not being adequately utilized, primarily attributable to pediatricians' lack of training in prevention sciences, their discomfort in discussing sexuality and the brevity of office visits. Clearly, training health care providers in prevention science theory and skills and providing incentives to counsel their adolescent patients is an area that requires greater attention.

Community-level Interventions for Adolescents may be an Effective HIV Prevention Strategy

Most HIV interventions for adolescents operate at the individual or group-level, with high relapse rates even with short term follow-up. On a broader scale, community-level interventions are needed which create an atmosphere supportive of prevention norms by reinforcing HIV prevention messages (Coates, 1990; Kelly & Murphy, 1992). Community-level interventions may therefore sustain the initial adoption of HIV- preventive behaviours and, hopefully, amplify programme effects over an extended follow-up period.

Community-level interventions designed to promote behaviour change are aimed at providing adolescents with information and skills to change behaviour through naturally occurring channels of influence in the community, and simultaneously to provide a supportive environment that encourages health-promoting behaviour change. Changing community norms also reinforces and maintains the practice of health-promoting behaviours. This provides one avenue for ensuring a context in which adolescents will be reminded that the healthier alternative is preferred according to community standards and norms. While community-level interventions are a promising intervention strategy, their effectiveness has not been empirically substantiated.

Tailoring HIV- Prevention Programmes to be Culturally, Developmentally and Gender-appropriate

Adolescents are not a homogeneous population, but rather a mosaic of sub-groups, each with differing subcultural values and norms. As such, the HIV epidemic among adolescents is not a unitary epidemic, but many epidemics, each differentially impacting selected adolescent populations. Thus, HIV- prevention programmes need to acknowledge this diversity between adolescent subgroups and include specific intervention strategies that are tailored to meet the needs of diverse adolescent populations. "Tailoring" would include assuring that interventions are culturally-sensitive, developmentally-appropriate and gender-relevant (Wingood & DiClemente, 1992, 1995; Airhihenbuwa *et al.*, 1992; Fullilove *et al.*, 1990).

Public and Healthy Policy: The Role of "Preventive Synergy"

The impact of any singular intervention strategy promoting the adoption and maintenance of HIV- preventive behaviour among adolescents should not be exaggerated. Single intervention strategies alone will not achieve maximal effectiveness if adolescents live in environments that regularly counteract newly acquired HIV- prevention knowledge and skills. Needed is "preventive synergy". Preventive synergy is the cumulative reinforcement of messages using co-ordinated, diverse intervention channels and resources. Such redundancy through manifold channels may lead to change whereas any single message delivered through a single channel may be insufficient to motivate behaviour change.

A related concept is "interdigitation of prevention resources". In essence, a need exists to link HIV- prevention resources into a network. This network, for example, would consist of community, schools, health providers, local government agencies and non-governmental agencies or community-based organizations. The role of this network would be to provide a web of preventive resources supporting reinforcement of prevention messages and linkage with health care systems. For example, multiple access points (i.e., recreation centers, after-school programmes, and physicians' offices) could be utilized as opportunity sites for providing HIV-prevention information and teaching relevant health-promotion skills.

Dissemination of Effective HIV Prevention Interventions

Successfully confronting the challenge of HIV will require that research interventions are conducted on a scale broad enough to yield direct public health benefits (Kelly *et al.,* 1993). Ultimately, preventing HIV infections will not only depend on the development and evaluation of innovative behaviour change approaches, but also on how effectively experimental interventions can be translated and integrated into self-sustaining components of school curricula or community programmes (Peterson & DiClemente, 1994), particularly in those countries and adolescent subgroups most adversely impacted by the HIV epidemic. While the continued efforts of prevention scientists need to be directed at developing more effective HIV prevention interventions, existing interventions that have demonstrated programmatic efficacy need to be adequately disseminated. Future research efforts must also be directed at identifying mechanisms for the timely translation of existing effective intervention programmes for other countries.

Looking Forward: Future Directions for HIV Prevention

Future HIV- prevention intervention programmes must build on their historical roots. Programmes must be developed and evaluated on an ongoing basis to monitor programmatic efficacy; not only by measuring statistically significant self-reported changes in risk behaviours, but more meaningful changes as well, such as changes in the incidence of disease. Whenever possible, however, additional outcome measures which avoid adolescents' self-reports of behaviour change need to be included in the evaluation of interventions. In some cases, HIV incidence rates, over time, can serve as one index of programme efficacy. In many countries and in many adolescent subgroups, the incidence of HIV infections may not be a suitable outcome measure. In these instances, other surrogate biological markers, such as sexually transmitted diseases and indicators of related preventive behaviours, for example, possession of condoms or bleach and clean injection needles should be employed in behaviour change interventions. Programmes must also be modified according to evaluation feedback, thus, further refining the intervention and strengthening its potential to effectively promote behaviour change. And, as important as programme development is the need for effective channels of programme dissemination. Programmes which are evaluated and identified as effective should be widely disseminated through diverse channels and training provided to indigenous personnel to encourage the adoption and appropriate use of these intervention programmes. And, finally, for HIV- prevention interventions to progress more rapidly, a comprehensive and coordinated infrastructure to conceptualize, stimulate and support the continuum of intervention research necessary to control the HIV epidemic is still of critical importance (Coates, 1990). It must become clear that an international, cooperative effort is necessary to control the HIV epidemic. From nations which have already witnessed the suffering and death of thousands of adolescents to AIDS to those nations where HIV is still uncommon among adolescents, there is a growing awareness of the global scope of the problem and a willingness to commit resources to confront the epidemic. International organizations such as the World Health Organization (WHO) and the United States Centers for Disease Control and Prevention (CDC) are establishing collaborative disease surveillance and educational programmes.

CONCLUSION

In conclusion, while systematic HIV prevention programmes, adequately funded and innovative in design, offer the potential to effectively reduce adolescents' HIV-associated risk behaviours, these changes will not be radical nor swift. HIV behaviour change will not be realized as a result of a single, static intervention administered at one time point, but rather, programme effectiveness is enhanced when applied and evaluated continuously over an extended time period. Further, to increase the comprehension and, perhaps effectiveness of HIV- prevention programmes, they must be developed to be age-specific, culturally-sensitive, and gender-relevant. Clearly, if we are to successfully confront the challenge of HIV, prevention intervention programmes will play a major role.

REFERENCES

D'Angelo, L. & DiClemente, R.J. (1996) Sexually Transmitted Diseased and Human Immunodeficiency Virus Infection among Adolescents (in press). In DiClemente, R.J., Hansen, W., & Ponton, L. (Eds.) *Handbook of Adolescent Risk Behaviour.* New York, NY: Plenum Publishing Corp. In Press.

Aggleton P, O'Reilly K, Slutkin G, Davies P (1994) Risking everything? Risk behaviour, behaviour change, and AIDS. *Science*, **265**, 341-345.

Airhihenbuwa, C.O., DiClemente, R.J., Wingood, G.M. & Lowe, A. (1992) HIV/AIDS education and prevention among African-Americans: A focus on culture. *Journal of AIDS Education and Prevention*, **4**, 251-260.

American Academy of Pediatrics Committee on Adolescence (1990) Contraception and adolescents. *Pediatrics*, **86**, 134-138.

Bandura, A. (1994). Social cognitive theory and exercise of control over HIV infection. In DiClemente, R.J., & Peterson, J. (Eds). Preventing AIDS: Theories and Methods of Behavioural Interventions. New York, NY: Plenum Publishing Corp; 25-59.

Bandura, A. (1992) A social cognitive approach to the exercise of control over AIDS infection. In DiClemente, R.J. (Ed.) Adolescents and AIDS: A generation in jeopardy. Newbury Park, Ca: Sage Publishing Company; 89-116.

Botvin, G. (1986) Substance abuse prevention research: Recent developments and future directions. *Journal of School Health*, **56**, 369-373.

Choi, K.H. & Coates, T.J. (1994) Prevention of HIV infection. *AIDS*, **8**, 1371-1389.

Coates, T.J. (1990) Strategies for modifying sexual behaviour for primary and secondary prevention of HIV disease. *Journal of Consulting and Clinical Psychology*, **58**, 57-69.

DiClemente, R.J., Zorn, J., & Temoshok, L. (1986) Adolescents' and AIDS: A survey of knowledge, beliefs and attitudes about AIDS in San Francisco. *American Journal of Public Health*, **76**, 1443-1445.

DiClemente, R.J. & Houston-Hamilton, A. (1989) Strategies for prevention of Human Immunodeficiency Virus infection among minority adolescents. *Health Education*, **20**, 39-43.

DiClemente, R.J. (1991) Predictors of HIV- preventive sexual behaviour in a high-risk adolescent population: The influence of perceived peer norms and sexual communication on incarcerated adolescents' consistent use of condoms. *Journal of Adolescent Health*, **12**, 385-390.

DiClemente, R.J. (1992) Psychosocial determinants of condom use among adolescents. In DiClemente, R.J. (Ed.), Adolescents and AIDS: A generation in jeopardy. Newbury Park, CA:Sage Publications, Inc, 34-51.

DiClemente, R.J. (1993) Confronting the challenge of AIDS among adolescents: Directions for future research. *Journal of Adolescent Research*, **8**, 156-166.

DiClemente, R.J. (1993) Preventing HIV/AIDS among adolescents: Schools of agents of change. *Journal of the American Medical Association*, **270**, 760-762.

DiClemente, R.J., & Brown, L.K. (1994) Expanding the pediatrician's role in HIV prevention for adolescents. *Clinical Pediatrics*, **32**, 235-240.

DiClemente, R.J., & Peterson, J. (1994) Changing HIV/AIDS risk behaviours: The role of behavioural interventions. In DiClemente, R.J., & Peterson, J. (Eds). *Preventing AIDS: Theories and methods of behavioural interventions*. New York, NY: Plenum Publishing Corporation; 1-4.

DiClemente, R.J., Lodico, M., Grinstead, O.A. Harper, G., Rickman, R.L., Evans, P.E. & Coates, T.J. (in press) African-American adolescents residing in high-risk urban environments do use condoms: Correlates and predictors of condom use among adolescents in public housing developments. *Pediatrics.*

DiClemente, R.J., & Houston-Hamilton, A. (1989) Strategies for prevention of Human Immunodeficiency Virus infection among minority adolescents. *Health Education*, **20**, 39-43.

DiClemente, R.J., & Brown, L.K. (1994) Expanding the Pediatrician's role in HIV prevention for adolescents. *Clinical Pediatrics.* **32**, 1-6.

Fisher, J.D. & Fisher, W.A. (1992) Changing AIDS-related risk behaviour. *Psychological Bulletin*, **111**, 455-474.

Fullilove, M.T., Fullilove, R., Bowser, B.P., Haynes, K., & Gross S.A. (1990) Black women and AIDS: Gender rules. *Journal of Sex Research*, **27**, 47-64.

Grimley, D., DiClemente, R.J. Prochaska, J.O., & Riley, G. (1995) Application of the Transtheoretical Model to preventing pregnancy, STDs, and HIV among adolescents. *Family Life Educator*, Spring, 7-15.

Hansen, W.B. & Graham, J.W. (1991) Preventing alcohol, marijuana and cigarette use among adolescents: Peer pressure resistance training versus establishing conservative norms. *Preventive Medicine*, **20**, 414-430.

Joffe, A. (1993) Adolescents and condom use. *American Journal of Diseases of Children*, **147**, 746-754.

Kelly, J.A., St. Lawrence, J.S., Diaz, Y.E. *et al.* (1991) HIV risk behaviour reduction following intervention with key opinion leaders of population: An experimental analysis. *American Journal of Public Health*, **81**, 168-171.

Kelly, J.A. & Murphy, D.A. (1992) Psychological interventions with AIDS and HIV: Prevention and treatment. *Journal of Consulting and Clinical Psychology*, **60**, 476-485.

Kelly, J.A. Murphy, D.A., Sikkemas, K.J., Kalichman, S.C. (1993) Psychological interventions are urgently needed to prevent HIV infection: New priorities for behavioural research in the second decade of AIDS. *American Psychologist*, **48**, 1023-1034.

Kirby, D. & DiClemente, R.J. (1994) School-based interventions to prevent unprotected sex and HIV among adolescents. In DiClemente, R.J. & Peterson, J. (Eds). Preventing AIDS: Theories and Methods of Behavioural Interventions, New York, NY: Plenum Publishing Corp; 117-139.

Klepp, K.I., Halper, A., & Perry, C.L. (1986) The efficacy of peer leaders in drug abuse prevention. *Journal of School Health*, **56**, 407-411.

Perry, C.L., & Grant, M. (1988) Comparing peer-led to teacher-led youth alcohol education in four countries. *Alcohol Health Research World*, **12**, 322-326.

Perry, C.L., & Sieving, R. (1993) Peer involvement in global AIDS prevention among Unpublished Manuscript.

Peterson, J.L., & DiClemente, R.J. (1994) Lessons Learned from Behavioural Interventions: Caveats, Gaps and Implications. In: DiClemente, R.J., & Peterson, J.L. (Eds.), Preventing AIDS: Theories and methods of behavioural interventions. New York, NY: Plenum Publishing Corporation; 319-321.

Prochaska, J.O., & DiClemente, C.C. (1983) Stages and processes of self-change in smoking: Toward an integrative model of change. *Journal of Consulting and Clinical Psychology*. **5**, 390-395.

Prochaska, J.O., & DiClemente, C.C. (1984) *The transtheoretical approach: Crossing the traditional boundaries of therapy*. Homewood, IL: Dow Jones/Irwin.

Rickert, V.I., Jay, M.S., Gottlieb, A., & Bridges, C. (1989) Adolescents and AIDS. Female attitudes and behaviours toward condom purchase and use. *Journal of Adolescent Health Care*, **10**, 313-316.

Robinson, T.N. Killen, J.D., Taylor, B., et al. (1987) Perspectives on adolescent substance abuse. *Journal of the American Medical Association*, **258**, 2072-2076.

Slap, G.B. Plotkin, S.L., Khalid, N., Michelman, D.F., & Forke, C.M. (1991) A human immunodeficiency virus peer education program for adolescent females. *Journal of Adolescent Health*, **12**, 434-442.

Telch, M.J. Miller, L.M. Killen, J.D., Cooke, S., et al. (1990) Social influences approach to smoking prevention: The effects of videotape delivery with and without same-age peer leader participation. *Addictive Behaviour*, **15**, 21-28.

Wight, D. (1992) Impediments to safer heterosexual sex: A review of research with young people. *AIDS Care*, **4**, 11-21.

Wingood, G.M. & DiClemente, R.J. (1992) Cultural, gender and psychological influences on HIV- related behaviour of African-American female adolescents: Implications for the development of tailored prevention programs. *Ethnicity & Disease*, **2**, 381-388.

Wingood, G.M. & DiClemente, R.J. (1995) Understanding the role of gender relations in HIV prevention research. *American Journal of Public Health*, **85**, 592.

Index

For Product Safety Concerns and Information please contact our EU representative GPSR@taylorandfrancis.com Taylor & Francis Verlag GmbH, Kaufingerstraße 24, 80331 München, Germany